D1216124

HANDBOOK OF PSYCHOSOCIAL NURSING CARE

EX LIBRIS

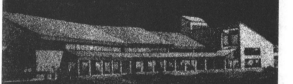

THE EDWARD AND DORIS MORTOLA LIBRARY

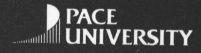

PACE
UNIVERSITY

PLEASANTVILLE, NEW YORK

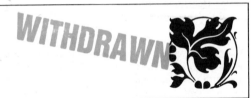

HANDBOOK OF PSYCHOSOCIAL NURSING CARE

CAROL REN KNEISL
R.N., M.S.

HOLLY SKODOL WILSON
R.N., Ph.D, F.A.A.N.

ADDISON-WESLEY PUBLISHING COMPANY
NURSING DIVISION ■ Menlo Park, California
Reading, Massachusetts ■ London ■ Amsterdam
Don Mills, Ontario ■ Sydney

Sponsoring Editor: Thomas Eoyang
Production Editor: Betty Duncan-Todd
Book Designer: Janet Bollow
Cover Designer: Don Taka
Copy Editor: Judith LaVigna

Copyright © 1984 by Addison-Wesley Publishing Company, Inc.
All rights reserved. No part of this publication may be
reproduced, stored in a retrieval system, or transmitted, in
any form or by any means, electronic, mechanical,
photocopying, recording, or otherwise, without the prior
permission of the publisher. Printed in the United States
of America. Published simultaneously in Canada.

Library of Congress Cataloging in Publication Data

Kneisl, Carol Ren, 1938-
    Handbook of psychosocial nursing care.
    1. Psychiatric nursing—Handbooks, manuals, etc.
2. Psychology, Pathological—Handbooks, manuals, etc.
3. Sick—Psychology—Handbooks, manuals, etc. I. Wilson,
Holly Skodol. II. Title. [DNLM: 1. Psychiatric nursing—
Handbooks. 2. Nurse-Patient relations—Handbooks.
3. Nursing assessment—Handbooks. WY 39 K68h]
RC440.K56   1984   610.73'68   84-478
ISBN 0-201-11705-3
    BCDEFGHIJ-KP-8987654

The authors and publishers have exerted every effort to
ensure that drug selection, dosage, and composition of
formulas set forth in this text are in accord with current
formulations, recommendations, and practice at the time of
publication. However, in view of ongoing research,
changes in government regulations, the reformulation of
nutritional products, and the constant flow of information
relating to drug therapy and drug reactions, the reader is
urged to check product information on composition or the
package insert for each drug for any change in indications
of dosage and for added warnings and precautions. This is
particularly important where the recommended agent is a
new and/or infrequently employed drug.

Addison-Wesley Publishing Company
Nursing Division
2725 Sand Hill Road
Menlo Park, California 94025

Ref
RC
470
. K56
1984

PREFACE

PURPOSE

Whether in private practice, community programs, psychiatric or general hospitals or clinics, nurses concern themselves with holistic human responses to health and illness. Whatever the setting or client group, nurses must know something—perhaps a great deal—about the psychosocial care of their clients. They must be able to assess, for instance, whether a confused elderly person is admitted to the emergency room because of substance abuse, a neurologic disease, schizophrenia, or other cause. They must be ready to intervene with clients in panic or those who threaten suicide. They must be able to evaluate responses of children at various developmental levels to the experience of hospitalization or of painful, intrusive procedures. In short, psychosocial care is a basic component of all nursing care, regardless of specialty area, primary diagnosis, or the client's location in the health care system.

The *Handbook of Psychosocial Nursing Care* is designed for the nurse who needs uncomplicated, ready access to essential information on psychosocial assessment and intervention strategies. Its small size, alphabetical organization, and emphasis on practical information make it easy to carry and use in any clinical setting for decision making and charting. It can be used in conjunction with our textbook, *Psychiatric Nursing,* Second Edition (Addison-Wesley, 1983) when the nurse requires additional understanding of the theoretic rationale underlying actions. When used alone, however, it eliminates the need to sift through a large, comprehensive textbook that may not be available when a clinical decision must be made on the spot.

FEATURES

This handbook gathers together the "how-to's" of clinical psychosocial nursing care. Its organization includes the following special features:

- An alphabetical format making problems or topics easy to locate
- Definitions of key terminology
- Assessment and intervention guidelines for major psychosocial client problems
- Lists, charts, tables, and sample nursing care plans stressing application of information and principles
- Thorough cross-referencing throughout
- Current DSM-III psychiatric diagnostic categories, criteria, and nomenclature
- Extensive Appendices on Psychotropic and Recreational Drugs, the 1982 ANA Standards of Psychiatric and Mental Health Nursing Practice, and all five axes of the American Psychiatric Association's 1980 DSM III.

For additional ease of access to pertinent information, the reader can use the inside covers to locate tables and entries that contain specific nursing interventions.

AUDIENCE

We believe this handbook can refresh and update practicing nurses who learned the processes and principles of psychosocial care earlier in their careers. It also responds to the expressed need of students and new graduates who must apply the nursing process to clients whose nursing diagnoses include psychosocial needs and problems. The *Handbook of Psychosocial Nursing Care* is portable, progressive, pertinent, professional, and practical. It should be a valuable adjunct to comprehensive nursing textbooks used in nursing programs, particularly when psychosocial concepts are valued as essential to the nurse's clinical repertoire with all clients.

ACKNOWLEDGMENTS

In addition to new content prepared especially for this volume, we have also drawn upon the second edition of our text, *Psychiatric Nursing*. Our own chapters and those of our contributors have been reformatted, reshaped, or reworked to meet the specific goals of this handbook. Some of its substance reflects the work and the ideas of Pamela Burton, Carol Bradley Corpuel, Priscilla Ebersole, Joanne Keglovits, Beth Moscato, Joan Sayre, Andrew E. Skodol, Patricia R. Underwood, Mary-Eve Mirenda Zangari. We appreciate the help of Cheryl Laskowski who helped to identify and compile content from *Psychiatric Nursing* to be included here.

Carol Ren Kneisl
Holly Skodol Wilson

CONTENTS

TABLES

NURSING INTERVENTIONS

Nursing Interventions included under these entries:

APPENDICES

A

ACTING OUT

The expression of unconscious conflicts through behavior; the unconscious impulse is not verbalized or remembered.

Acting out is a form of resistance in which the client puts into action a memory that has been forgotten or repressed. The client's conflict is thus externalized and always involves other people in the environment. Acting out is difficult to deal with because the client does not talk about the feelings that precipitate the behavior and later tends to conceal or rationalize the behavior. Acting out can abruptly break up treatment unless it is identified and dealt with explicitly.

(*See also* Resistance; Transference)

ACUTE INTERMITTENT PORPHYRIA

Disorders involving the substance porphyrin, which is involved in cellular metabolism throughout the body. They are commonly misdiagnosed because of their unusual and varied clinical presentations. This relatively rare disease may affect several members of the same family. Classically, females are more affected than males.

Assessment

- Attacks, characterized by abdominal pain, are induced by ingestion of certain kinds of drugs, including barbiturates, alcohol, and sulfa drugs.
- Hypertension, photosensitive skin, peripheral neuropathy, and muscle wasting are physical signs.
- A wide variety of behaviors mimicking neurotic and psychotic states may occur during an attack.

Medical Treatment

- chlorpromazine (Thorazine) for abdominal pain
- prophylactic avoidance of precipitating drugs

(*See also* Organic Brain Syndrome)

ADDICTED LIFE STYLES
Disruptive life style having complex physiologic, psychologic, and sociologic dimensions. (Categorized in DSM III as a personality disorder on Axis II.)

(*See also* Alcohol/Alcoholic/Alcoholism; Personality Disorders; Substance Use Disorders)

ADDICTION
Strong dependence, both physiologic and emotional, on alcohol or some other drug. The term *drug dependence* is gradually replacing *drug addiction*.

(*See also* Substance Use Disorders)

ADDISON'S DISEASE
Adrenal cortical insufficiency that may cause organic mental changes that are largely affective (anxiety or depression) or frankly psychotic.

Assessment

- Symptoms include anorexia, weight loss, nausea, vomiting, and diarrhea.
- A classic sign is a bluish hyperpigmentation of skin and buccal mucosa.
- Hypoglycemia, electrolyte disturbances, and hypotension complicate adrenal crises.

Treatment

- Depends on the cause of the decrease in adrenal steroid output (bacterial or fungal infection, surgical removal, hemorrhage, or systemic disease such as amyloidosis or scleroderma) and the extent of the damage that has occurred before detection.

(*See also* Endocrine Disorders; Organic Brain Syndrome)

ADOLESCENCE
A stormy period in life characterized by rapid physical and sexual growth; frequently accompanied by conflicting ideas and feelings, it is an interruption between the docility of the latency years and the acclimation of adulthood.

CHARACTERISTICS

- Spectacular physical and sexual changes
- Gain in intellectual capacity and power, particularly in ability to form concepts, generalize, and abstract
- Increasing importance of peer relationships
- Emotional lability with doubts, uncertainties, and fears
- Identity versus role confusion (psychosocial task of early adolescence)
- Intimacy versus isolation (psychosocial task of late adolescence)

PROBLEM BEHAVIORS OF ADOLESCENTS

- Tend to be defiant, sullen, or flippant
- Often reluctant to talk about themselves
- Tend to engage in sexual acting out
- Often use alcohol or drugs for recreational purposes
- Frequently test authority and break rules
- May manipulate others
- Frequently bow to peer pressure
- May express anxiety, depression, feelings of infe-

riority, hostility, or self-destructive behavior
resulting from struggle with establishing identity

Nursing Intervention

- Assist adolescent to master current developmental
  stage and to progress to next.
- Avoid being judgemental, authoritarian, or
  punitive.
- Set rational and consistent limits on acting-out
  behavior.
- Provide opportunities for peer group interaction.

ADULT EGO STATE

In transactional analysis theory, the ego state responsible for the objective appraisal of reality and the
capacity to process data.

(*See also* Transactional Analysis)

AFFECT

Emotion or feeling; the tone of one's reaction to persons
and events.

Examples of disturbed affect include:

- *Blunted affect.* A dulling in the intensity of feeling
- *Flat affect.* A dull or blunt emotional tone attached
  to an object, idea, or thought (most frequently
  observed in schizophrenic disorders)
- *Inappropriate affect.* A response to an event, situation, or interaction that is inconsistent with the
  stimulus
- *Labile affect.* Abrubt, rapid, and repeated changes
  in affect for no apparent reason

AFFECTIVE DISORDER

Disturbed personal coping pattern in which the client
feels extreme sadness, withdraws socially, often feels

guilty, and expresses self-deprecatory thoughts or experiences an elevated expansive mood with hyperactivity, pressure of speech, inflated self-esteem, decreased need for sleep. These mood disturbances may occur alone or together and may show varying patterns of severity and duration.

(*See also* Bipolar Affective Disorder; Depressive Disorder)

AGED PERSONS

The onset of old age is generally believed to occur around the age of 70. Associated physical and psychologic changes vary among individuals. The following assessment tools may be used when working with elderly clients.

QUESTIONS TO PROMOTE PERSONAL REVELATION AMONG THE AGED

1. What are your areas of daily gratification? (Awareness of the present provides daily satisfaction.)
2. Who provides you with the greatest comfort and support? (Confidantes and intimates are essential to mental health.)
3. What experiences have had the most profound influence on you? (The past continues to influence our present abilities and expectations.)
4. What has been your most difficult experience and how did you handle it? (One's capacity for survival builds self-esteem.)
5. What unfulfilled hopes do you have? (Hope is essential to survival.)
6. What is your greatest problem right now? (Mutual problem solving creates an alliance of concern and promotes growth.)

GUIDELINES FOR ASSESSING THE SEXUAL NEEDS OF THE AGED

1. When you were growing up, did people you knew discuss sex and romance?

2. How do you feel about discussing sex and romance now?

3. What do you think about romance at this stage in your life?

4. What were you told about sex when you were a child?

5. Do you think sex is a very important part of life satisfaction for people of all ages?

6. How important has sexual activity been in your life?

7. What were you told about masturbation?

8. What does sexuality mean to you?

9. Does your present living situation give you opportunities to express your sexuality?

10. What values and morals influence your feelings about sex now?

11. How are your needs for intimacy being met now?

Drugs used by the aged may create various physical and emotional symptoms.

Drugs	Symptoms*
Hypoglycemics; hypotensives (phenothiazines, antidepressants, narcotic analgesics, antiarrhythmic drugs antihypertensives)	Nervousness, apprehension, irritability, disorientation, dizziness, syncope
Cortisone	Severe depression
Reserpine	Anxiety, depression, nightmares, orthostatic hypotension, Parkinsonian syndrome
Digitalis	Arrhythmias, confusion, agitation, disorientation, dizziness, apathy,

Drugs	Symptoms*
	depression, headache, hallucinations
Central nervous system depressants (major and minor tranquilizers, sedatives, hypnotics, alcohol, methyldopa, antidepressants, narcotic analgesics, resperine)	Lethargy, memory problems, perceptual disorders, delusions, agitation, panic, confusion
Anticholinergics (atropine, major tranquilizers, antidepressants, anti-Parkinsonian drugs)	Confusion, blurred vision, agitation, disorientation, impaired memory
Propranolol	Nightmares
Quinidine	Vertigo, tinnitus, headache
Procainamide	Manic behavior, giddiness, psychosis, hallucinations, depression
Lithium	Blurred vision, slurred speech, ataxia, tremors

*Data from Todd, B., Drugs and the elderly: could your patient's confusion be caused by drugs? *Geriatric Nursing* (May/June 1981): 219-20.

Grief in the aged client occurs as the result of frequent losses. Characteristics and intervention strategies are listed in Table 1. (See page 8.)

Crisis Intervention Techniques for the Aged

1. Identify crisis the client is experiencing.
2. Maintain routine, and support usual habits that

TABLE 1. GRIEF IN AGED CLIENT

CHARACTERISTICS	INTERVENTIONS
1. Chronicity or grief overload arising from multiple, frequent losses	1. Identify number of losses and presence of grief and depression since the client may not recognize it. Encourage verbal review of the losses.
2. Regret for what cannot be undone	2. Review context of life situation that produces regret and/or guilt.
3. Premature grief for one's own death and separation from loved ones	3. Listen to expressions of grief, establish legacy, provides opportunities for intimate time with loved ones, singly rather than in groups.
4. Grief for the alteration of one's own personality and cognition through disease processes	4. Support individual and family in focusing on remaining strengths and exchanging caring gestures.

5. Grief for loss of companionship with a mentally deteriorating aged spouse

5. Assist functioning spouse to establish or find a support group of persons in similar situation. Locate respite services for functioning spouse. Provide anticipatory guidance for handling problems of deterioration.

6. Survival anguish, particularly that of outliving children or siblings

6. Provide consistent support through grief process, paying particular attention to holidays and anniversary dates. Reduce survivor guilt by conducting life review and establishing legacy of the deceased.

7. Grief over the loss of body function or parts

7. Encourage mourning; do not avoid talking of the loss. Indicate that grief process is normal and painful. Listen. Help identify compensatory functions when acute grief subsides.

9

give a sense of security (familiar setting, cup of tea).

3. Review and clarify cognitive perception of the disruptive event.

4. Encourage reminiscing to learn client's characteristic behavior, level of self-esteem, past coping patterns, and unique needs.

5. Encourage expression of feelings to reduce anxiety and restore a sense of control.

6. Do not dismiss any complaint as unimportant.

7. Identify available supports for the client.

8. Write down or repeat important information as necessary.

9. Recognize the ruminative tendency during crises as necessary for restored function. Support this process by indicating to client that it is a stage in the resolution of crises.

10. Leave the client with some tangible benefit and a sense of hope (a phone number to call for assistance or a plan of action).

(*See also* Confusion; Appendix **B,** Principles of Administering Psychotropic Drugs to the Aged)

AGGRESSION

Forceful, goal-directed behavior that may be physical or verbal.

Nursing Intervention (physical aggression)

1. Address, rather than avoid, client's specific behavior. (Interrupts dysfunctional behavioral pattern)

2. Avoid retaliatory actions. (Retaliatory actions do not meet client's needs in a growth-facilitating manner)

3. Approach client in a calm, firm manner. (Provides role model of appropriate self-control)

4. Attempt to talk with client; convey acceptance of client but not of aggressive behavior. (Emphasizes

need to change behavioral pattern while maintaining positive regard for client)

5. Encourage alternative expressions of aggression such as use of foam bats or pillows. (Constructive channelings of energies teaches coping skills)

6. Intervene early when client gives first signs of aggression: frowns, threats, clenching of fists.

7. When necessary, remove client from immediate environment to help re-establish self-control. (Sets external limits until client can assume responsibility for self-control)

Nursing Intervention (verbal aggression)

1. Continue rather than avoid client contact. (Interrupts dysfunctional behavioral pattern)

2. Explore threat or frustration that preceded indication of hostility. (Focuses on thinking, rather than action and encourages identification of feelings)

3. Allow time and space for client to verbalize feelings (helplessness, inadequacy, anger) associated with threat or frustration. (New experience may be laden with anxiety)

4. Encourage client to make connections between specific threat or frustration, subsequent feelings, and specific manifestation of hostility. (Allows analysis of client's mode of conflict resolution)

5. Explore client's possible need for external controls such as medication or exercise; assess degree of closeness tolerated by client. (Sets limits regarding threatened aggressive contact)

6. Provide consistent set of expectations about and guidance toward self-control. (Respects personal choice, yet emphasizes expectation for self-control)

AKATHISIA

A reversible extrapyramidal syndrome characterized by motor restlessness experienced by the client as an urge to pace, a need to shift weight from one foot to the other, or an inability to sit or stand still. Responds well to oral antiparkinsonian agents. Akathisia may be confused with a psychotic relapse. The following list* differentiates the two.

Akathisia	Agitation or Relapse
Motor restlessness predominates, verbal complaints minimal	Verbalization prominent
Outside voluntary control	Controllable
Worsened by medication increase	Improved by medication increase
Reduction of phenothiazine relieves symptoms	Reduction of phenothiazine worsens symptoms
Responsive to anti-parkinsonian agents	Unresponsive to anti-parkinsonian agents

*Source: Adapted from Appleton, W.S., and Davis, J.M., 1973. *Practical Clinical Psychopharmacology.* Baltimore: Medcom, Inc., p. 57. The Williams & Wilkins Co., Baltimore.

(*See also* Appendix **B,** Antiparkinsonian Drugs)

ALCOHOL/ALCOHOLIC/ALCOHOLISM
Alcohol is a mind- and mood-altering substance, ingested as a liquid, and classified as a central nervous system depressant. Its consumption may have no apparent effect on the drinker. At moderate levels, it may produce euphoria; at high levels, it acts as a sedative. An intoxicating beverage is one that produces a blood-level concentration of alcohol of 0.10% or more. This concentration is the legal test for inebriation in many states.

Alcoholism is substance abuse combined with physical addiction. The term alcoholic is applied to those whose continued or excessive drinking results in impairment of personal health, disruption of family and social relationships, and loss of economic security.

PHYSIOLOGIC ACTION OF ALCOHOL

- Absorbed in small intestine
- 2-10% excreted through lungs, kidneys, and skin
- Remainder broken down in liver
- Acts as central nervous system depressant
- Stimulating qualities felt as result of release of inhibition
- In large doses acts as a severe depressant of respiratory centers
- Simple intoxication does not last longer than 12 hours and is usually followed by a hangover

MAJOR ILLNESSES ASSOCIATED WITH LONG-TERM USE OF ALCOHOL

- Alcoholic hepatitis
- Chronic gastritis
- Anemia
- Wernicke-Korsakoff syndrome (amnesia, confabulation, disorientation, peripheral neuropathy, clouding of consciousness, and sometimes coma)
- Peripheral neuropathy
- Beriberi
- Pellagra
- Laennec's cirrhosis
- Alcoholic cerebellar degeneration

Assessment

ACUTE PHASE OF ALCOHOL TOXICITY

The nurse usually encounters alcoholics first when they are acutely ill from the toxic effects of the drug and require hospitalization. The symptoms during this acute phase may include

1. Nausea and vomiting

2. Perspiration and weakness
3. Severe tremors, especially of hands and face
4. Myoclonic jerking of arms, legs, head, and neck, which may increase to the severity of generalized convulsions
5. Dilated pupils
6. Insomnia
7. Loss of appetite, or even inability to tolerate food
8. Dehydration
9. Slurred, often rambling and incoherent speech
10. Motor activity ranging from wild restlessness to a state of stupor
11. Emotional symptoms including anxiety, depression, irritability, hypersensitivity to light and sound, impaired memory, disorientation, inappropriate behavior, visual and auditory hallucinations, and impaired insight and judgment
12. Tendency to develop intercurrent respiratory infections, which may develop into pneumonia
13. Apparent poor hygiene and poor nutrition
14. If alcoholism is prolonged, nutritional and vitamin deficiencies, liver cirrhosis, chronic brain damage, and mental deterioration

ALCOHOL WITHDRAWAL SYMPTOMS

1. Tremors
2. Excessive perspiration
3. Nausea
4. Vomiting
5. Anorexia
6. Restlessness
7. Hallucinations
8. Convulsions
9. Delirium tremens

The nurse should determine if and what other drugs (prescription, over-the-counter, recreational) have been ingested by the individual. The reaction between alcohol and other substances may result in serious physical and mental impairment.

TABLE 2. ALCOHOL AND DRUG INTERACTIONS

Class (Generic Names)	General Effects	Specific Problems
Analgesics (aspirin, acetamino- phen)	Unpredictable	Delayed clotting time, gastro- intestinal bleeding, fecal blood loss, hemorrhage
Anesthetics (chloroform, ether)	Antagonistic, additive, supra-additive	Deep narcosis, excessive recovery time, more needed initially to induce sleep
Antialcohol preparations (disulfiram)	Untoward, life threatening	Increased blood pressure, facial flushing, tachycardia, headache, nausea, dizziness, fainting
Antianginal drugs, antihyperten- sives (nitroglycerin, methyldopa, hydralazine, guanethidine, reserpine) peripheral vasodilators	Antagonistic	Hypotension, faintness, loss of consciousness

(Continued)

15

TABLE 2. ALCOHOL AND DRUG INTERACTIONS (Continued)

Class (Generic Names)	General Effects	Specific Problems
Anti-convulsants (phenytoin)	Cross-tolerant	Accelerated metabolism, normal dosage inadequate
Anti-depressants (Monoamine-oxidase inhibitors)	Supra-additive, untoward, life threatening	Hypertensive crisis—particularly with Chianti wine and beer
Tricyclics	Antagonistic, additive	Increased susceptibility to convulsions; hypotension
Antidiabetics/hypoglycemics (tolbutamide, chlor-propamide, aceto-hexamide, tolazamide)	Unpredictable	Severe hypoglycemia, unpredictable fluctuations in serum glucose levels, increased rate of metabolism of drug
Antihistamines (diphen-hydramine)	Additive	Reduced performance ability; increased sedation, operation of machinery hazardous
Antimicrobials/anti-infectives (chlor-amphenicol, furazolidone, metronidazole,	Unpredictable	Similar to disulfiram reactions, but milder (see under antialcohol

TABLE 2. ALCOHOL AND DRUG INTERACTIONS (Continued)

Class (Generic Names)	General Effects	Specific Problems
griseofulvin, isoniazid, quinacrine)		preparations)
Barbiturates (secobarbital, pentobarbital)	Supra-additive, untoward, life threatening	Vomiting, severe motor impairment, unconsciousness, coma, and death
Chloral hydrate	Additive	Profound vasodilation—sometimes lasting 7 days after ingestion of alcohol; dysphoria, tachycardia
Minor tranquilizers (meprobamate, benzodiazepines, diazepam)	Supra-additive	Central nervous system depression, interference with skills and alertness; diazepam and alcohol combination is dangerous
Narcotics (meperidine, morphine, propoxyphene)	Additive, untoward, life threatening	Central nervous system depression
Stimulants (caffeine, amphetamine)	Antagonistic, additive, unpredictable	Variable effects on selected behaviors: *(Continued)*

TABLE 2. ALCOHOL AND DRUG INTERACTIONS (Continued)

Class (Generic Names)	General Effects	Specific Problems
		depression, released inhibitions

Modified from U.S. Department of Health, Education, and Welfare. 1979. *FDA Drug Bulletin.* 2. U.S. Government Printing Office.

Nursing Intervention

The primary goals of the nurse are to identify alcoholics and coordinate a system of treatment that includes crisis intervention or acute emergency care; detoxification; and medical or psychiatric inpatient followup care, halfway houses, and aftercare.

Treatment during the acute phase of alcoholism (also referred to as drying out or detoxification) usually occurs in a well-controlled environment such as a hospital. A number of support measures are directed toward relieving symptoms.

- Some type of sedation or tranquilizer
- Medication to relieve symptoms of nausea and insomnia
- Adequate diet
- Replacement fluids
- Vitamin therapy
- Antibiotics if infections are present
- Some tranquilizers to control uncooperative behavior

During the recovery phase of alcoholism, several therapeutic conditions are important for success.

- Group therapy and/or involvement in a support group
- Family involvement in long-range treatment plan

- Followup care
- Therapist availability at critical times

  Measures for preventing alcoholism include:

- Training people to tolerate increased stress and to learn improved coping patterns
- Preparing people in advance for difficult or painful events
- Reducing irritating or frustrating environmental stress
- Reducing social isolation
- Attempting to alter alcoholic beverages chemically to lessen their addictive qualities
- Instituting measures to regulate the sale and distribution of alcoholic beverages
- Promoting educational programs in schools on the use and abuse of alcohol
- Finding substitute tension-reducing strategies

ALGORITHMS
Behavioral steps, or step-by-step procedures, for the management of common problems to provide structured, standardized guidelines for decision making.

(See Depressive Disorder for a sample algorithm)

ALZHEIMER'S DISEASE
Atrophy of the cerebral cortex that can begin at a relatively young age (40-60 years). The cause of this disease is unknown, and there is no known treatment.

Assessment

- Symptoms are characteristic of diseases affecting the cortex. Clients have problems with speech, motor coordination, recognition of familiar objects (even parts of their own bodies), and naming.

- Mental functions deteriorate slowly but progressively, leading to reduced intellectual capacity, impaired memory, loss of social sense, and apathy or restlessness. These may at first be mistaken for an involutional depression.
- Brain tests such as pneumoencephalograms reveal cortical atrophy.
- Seizures may complicate the picture.

(*See also* Organic Brain Syndrome)

AMBIVALENCE
The coexistence of positive and negative feelings about objects, events, situations, or interactions. These feelings produce the desire to do two opposite things at once.

AMNESIA
Sudden and total loss of memory for events of a period of time ranging from a few hours to a lifetime. Psychogenic amnesia is a dissociative disorder due to psychologic mechanisms. In localized amnesia, the most common form of psychogenic amnesia, a person loses memory only for specific and related past times, usually surrounding a disturbing event.

The following list compares dissociative (psychogenic) amnesia with postconcussional (traumatic injury) amnesia.

Dissociative Amnesia	Postconcussional Amnesia
No history of head injury	History of head injury
Retrograde amnesia extends indefinitely into the past	Retrograde amnesia does not extend beyond a week into the past
Client can recover suddenly with total	Amnesia disappears slowly and memory is not

Dissociative Amnesia	Postconcussional Amnesia
restoration of memory	completely restored for events that occurred during the amnesic period

AMPHETAMINE

A central nervous system stimulant. Amphetamines have effects similar to those of ephedrine: constriction of peripheral blood vessels, stimulation of heart and increased blood pressure, relaxation of bronchial and intestinal muscles, and decreased appetite. These drugs are used as mood elevators and appetite depressants. They are also used to combat drowsiness. As tolerance to these drugs develops, the sense of well-being is increasingly blurred by apprehension and increased emotional lability—particularly characterized by hostile impulsiveness. Withdrawal from amphetamines usually causes depression and somnolence.

(*See also* Drug Use)

AMYOTROPHIC LATERAL SCLEROSIS

A degenerative neurologic disease of unknown etiology, with an adult onset, that affects the pyramidal tracts of the spinal cord and results in abnormalities of motor function. Also known as Lou Gehrig's disease.

Assessment

- Cranial and spinal lower motor neurons may be affected leading to muscle weakness, atrophy, tremors, and diminished tone of the facial musculature and proximal extremities.
- Although cases of mental changes are somewhat rare, there are a significant number of reported dis-

turbances of mood, affect, social behavior, and reality testing associated with the disease.

(*See also* Organic Brain Syndrome)

ANA STANDARDS OF PSYCHIATRIC AND MENTAL HEALTH NURSING PRACTICE

(*See* Appendix **A**)

ANACLITIC DEPRESSION

Term used to describe infants separated from their mothers (or other primary caregivers) during the first year of life because of prolonged hospitalization of the child or placement in an institution such as an orphanage. These infants often become withdrawn, apathetic, and emaciated.

(*See also* Hospitalized Child)

ANOREXIA NERVOSA

A condition characterized by severe emaciation due to an intense fear of becoming obese and a disturbance in body image such that the individual feels fat even when grotesquely thin. Most reported cases occur in adolescent females.

Anorexia nervosa must be distinguished from weight loss seen in a number of psychiatric disturbances including:

1. Psychotic disorders (Agitation, apathy, or delusions about poisoning may be responsible for reduction in eating.)
2. Depression (General unhappiness results in loss of appetite.)
3. Geriatric states (Adjustment and adaptive problems may lead the elderly to give up good dietary practices.)
4. Psychogenic malnutrition

5. Obese adolescents with counterphobic behavior
6. Histrionic individuals with repressed and displaced sexual conflicts leading to difficulty in swallowing
7. Obsessional individuals with self-punitive behavior leading to starvation
8. Adolescent females with pregnancy fears

In anorexia nervosa, a major life change, such as the first sexual encounter or moving away from home, often precipitates the onset of the syndrome. Some clients merely take in less food while others eat but immediately self-induce vomiting (see bulimia). Typically the client's resolve falters after a time, and binge eating occurs. This invariably is followed by guilt and further dietary restriction or vomiting.

Assessment

Signs and symptoms associated with anorexia nervosa are:

1. Weight loss
2. Amenorrhea
3. Hyperactivity
4. Constipation
5. Hypotension
6. Bradycardia
7. Hypothermia
8. Hyperkeratosis of skin
9. Secondary sexual organ atrophy
10. Leukopenia
11. Anemia
12. Hypoglycemia
13. Hypercholesterolemia
14. Hypoproteinemia
15. Reduced basal metabolic rate
16. Reduced gonadotropins
17. Normal thyroid function

18. Normal adrenal cortical function

Nursing Intervention

Anorexia nervosa can develop into a life-threatening emergency. Up to 15% of those afflicted die of malnutrition, and another fraction are prone to suicide. Thus the nurse's consistent and constant attention to the client is necessary to ensure his or her well-being. The following are suggested interventions to be used in treatment of the client suffering from anorexia nervosa.

When the problem is ambivalence about food:

1. Set specific amount of time for eating.
2. Provide one-to-one supervision during meals at a table separate from other clients to observe closely for hiding of food.
3. Do not encourage client to eat.
4. Check tray to avoid omissions or substitutions.
5. After time limit is over, pick up tray without speaking to client about it.
6. Check for uneaten food, look under plates and napkins.
7. Give blended tube feedings if ordered.
8. Provide one-to-one supervision in dayroom area for 30 minutes after meals.
9. Bathroom privileges should be decided by staff; generally, withhold these immediately after eating. Supervise client for 30 minutes after meals.
10. Set limits on physical activity; chart activity level on the ward.
11. Weigh client three times weekly at specified time in only hospital gown and pajamas.

Outcome: Client will have adequate dietary intake for weight gain.

When the problem is anger at staff over loss of autonomy as a result of regimen restrictions:

1. One staff member should work with physician in planning consistent treatment regimen and presenting this to client.
2. Client's questions will be answered at initial presentation; later questions are to be directed to the physician.
3. Staff should not converse with client about food or weight.
4. Acknowledge client's anger when it is verbalized, but do not deal with issues of weight or food.
5. Staff must be consistent in all aspects of regimen.
6. Any staff member's questions about the regimen should be referred to team or client's nurse.

Outcome: The regimen will remain constant while anger and feeling of ineffectuality are acknowledged.

When the problem is cachexia, and/or malnourishment, and/or dehydration:

1. Discourage daily bathing.
2. Provide lanolin cream after bathing and twice a day.
3. Massage skin over bony prominences twice a day; teach patient to do likewise.
4. Carefully monitor vital signs.
5. Discourage use of laxatives.

Outcome: Client will be adequately hydrated; skin integrity will be maintained; vital signs will be clearly monitored as an aid in evaluating health status.

ANTICIPATORY GUIDANCE
A process that aims to help persons cope with a crisis by discussing the details of the impending difficulty and problem solving before the event occurs.

ANTIDEPRESSANT DRUG
A medication used to treat severe depression. Antidepressants are divided into two principal categories,

the tricyclic compounds and the monoamine oxidase inhibitors.

(*See also* Appendix **B,** Antidepressant Drugs)

ANTIPSYCHOTIC DRUG

A medication used to control certain psychotic symptoms, notably disordered thinking, agitation, and excitement. The principal classes of antipsychotics are phenothiazines, thioxanthenes, butyrophenones, and rauwolfias.

(*See also* Appendix **B,** Antipsychotic Drugs)

ANTISOCIAL PERSONALITY DISORDER

Characterized by behavior patterns that are in conflict with society, frequently including criminal or violent acts. Features include:

1. Normal feelings of deliberateness and intention are impaired. This impairment is manifested to the individual as an irresistible impulse. The whim is paramount.
2. Feelings are carried along by moment-to-moment events and significant actions are executed without a clear and complete sense of motivation, decision, or sustained wish.
3. When asked why they behaved as they did, they may say:
   —"I just felt like it;"
   —"I didn't want to do it, but somehow I just did;"
   —"I didn't really want to do it, but I just gave in;"
   —"I was just carried along by the events."
   All these explanations reflect an abrupt, transient, and partial experience of deciding in which the sense of active intention is impaired.
4. Action is rapid and abrupt without planning.

5. Poor judgment and a conspicuous lack of long-range planning are evident.
6. Moral values are underdeveloped and uninfluential; conscience is perfunctory.
7. Insincerity and lying are characteristic.
8. These persons see the world as a discontinuous inconstant composite of opportunities, temptations, frustrations, sensuous experiences, and fragmented impressions. They do not search beyond the immediately relevant present because their interests and emotional involvements are limited to immediate gains and satisfactions.

Nursing Intervention

Treatment is aimed at helping these clients control their behavior by maintaining a firm but accepting attitude toward them while imposing external limits on their actions. Often such a therapeutic plan is undertaken in a totally inpatient milieu. Nurses are most likely to encounter these clients in a correctional institution or general hospital.

The nurse who works with clients who have antisocial personality disorders needs to be:

1. Patient
2. Able to control personal resentment
3. Intuitive
4. Insightful
5. Warm without being seductive
6. Firm without being punitive
7. Able to accept the client's feelings without identifying with the modes of behavior
8. Able to use authority rationally and judiciously for the client's benefit
9. Able to give unconditionally
10. Able to accept the client's idiom and behavior without adopting them

11. Able to persevere kindly but tenaciously when faced with manipulation of limits
12. Able to tolerate verbal abuse from the client when enforcing limits

The general goals of treatment in the context of a one-to-one long-term relationship are to:

1. Provide a model of mature behavior
2. Develop a positive relationship
3. Mobilize some anxiety in the client while encouraging him or her to persist in the therapeutic relationship
4. Convey concern and interest in the client
5. Use problem-solving techniques to help the client make environmental changes, such as stable living arrangements and work plans
6. Encourage the client to inhibit acting-out behaviors and rely more on verbal communication, thereby enhancing both self-control and self-esteem
7. Help the client who has developed a more positive and realistic self-concept to continue the process of personal growth, which has usually been arrested in the preadolescent and adolescent years
8. Anticipate and deal with depression in clients who gradually develop enough insight to realize and accept responsibility for behavior that has injured others

(*See also* Personality Disorders)

ANXIETY

A diffuse feeling of dread, apprehension, or unexplained discomfort; a subjectively painful warning of impending danger that motivates the individual to take corrective action to relieve this unpleasant feeling.

DEGREES OF ANXIETY

Mild to moderate anxiety can be functionally effective in that it helps focus attention and generates energy and motivation. Severe anxiety and panic narrow attention to a crippling degree: Alertness is greatly reduced and learning does not usually take place. The following list further delineates levels of anxiety:

- *Mild anxiety.* Perceptual field is broad. Alertness is increased, observations are keen, connection between events is clear.
- *Moderate anxiety.* Perceptual field is narrowed. Alertness is increased, and concentration is centered on one specific thing. That which is irrelevant to the task or issue at hand is shut out (selective inattention). Connections between events are still understandable.
- *Severe anxiety.* Perceptual field is completely disrupted, with distortion and enlargement of a detail that previously served as a focal point. Most attempts to communicate are unintelligible to the listener. A *panic state* could be described as the disintegration of personality organization and control into innumerable bits. A person experiences this disintegration as the most intense terror.

SOURCES OF ANXIETY

People experience anxiety in many different kinds of situations and interpersonal relationships. The stimulus varies with the individual. However, the general causes of anxiety have been classified into two major kinds of threats:

1. Threats to biologic integrity: actual or impending interference with basic human needs such as the need for food, drink, or warmth

2. Threats to the security of self:
    a. unmet expectations important to self-integrity
    b. unmet needs for status and prestige
    c. anticipated disapproval by significant others
    d. inability to gain or reinforce self-respect or to gain recognition from others
    e. guilt, or discrepancies between self-view and actual behavior

Assessment

- Mild anxiety underlies such observable irritations as restlessness, sleeplessness, hostility, belittlings, misunderstandings, and the like. It also underlies persistent curiosity, repetitive questioning, constant attention seeking, and approval or reassurance seeking.
- Mild and moderate anxiety usually speed up physiological operations, whereas severe anxiety slows them down and can even paralyze them.
- Prolonged panic can result in a complete paralysis of functioning, culminating in death.

Nursing Care Plan for Anxious Client

Step of Plan	Nursing Intervention
1. Observe client for increased psychomotor activity, anger or withdrawal, excessive demands, and tearfulness.	Verbalizations intended to help client recognize and name his experience as anxiety: "Are you feeling uncomfortable?" "Are you anxious or nervous now?" When client says "Yes," he is ready for Step 2.
2. Connect feeling of anxiety with relief behavior. Client acknowledges,	Ask client what he does to feel more comfortable when he feels anxious. When client understands

Step of Plan	Nursing intervention
describes, and names feelings of nervousness or anxiety.	that when he feels anxious he gets angry, withdraws, or somatizes, he is ready for Step 3.
3. Investigate situation that immediately preceded feeling of anxiety.	Encourage client to recall and describe what he was experiencing immediately before he got anxious (including thoughts, actions, and other feelings).

4. Help client observe, describe, and analyze connections between what led to his anxiety and what happened after he felt anxious. Only through seeing all parts of this experience can client understand why he became anxious.

5. Formulate causes of anxiety. Help client state causes of the anxiety. Then help him observe and recall similar instances in his experiences of anxiety. Through such extensive discussions, client will eventually be able to recognize and perhaps alter his pattern of handling anxiety.

*Source: Peplau, H. "Interpersonal Techniques: The Crux of Nursing." Copyright © 1962. American Journal of Nursing Company. Adapted with permission from the *American Journal of Nursing,* June, Vol. 62 No. 6.

(*See also* Appendix **B,** Antianxiety Drugs)

Nursing Intervention for Client in Panic

1. Stay physically with client.
2. Maintain calm, serene manner.
3. Use short, simple sentences and firm, authoritative voice.
4. Encourage client to move to a smaller physical

environment, such as his or her room, to minimize the stimuli.

5. Sometimes it is useful to focus client's diffuse energy on some physically tiring task such as moving furniture or scrubbing the floor.

6. Consider recommending that antianxiety medication be ordered for client.

ANXIETY DISORDER

Disturbed personal coping pattern in which anxiety is either the predominant disturbance or a secondary disturbance that is confronted if the primary symptom is taken away.

The DSM III divides anxiety disorders into two types:

1. Panic disorder: characterized by sudden, intense, and discrete periods of extreme fear accompanied by symptoms such as dyspnea, palpitations, chest pain, choking sensations, dizziness, derealization, paresthesias, hot and cold flashes, sweating, faintness, trembling or shaking, and a fear of impending doom

2. Generalized anxiety disorder: manifested by steady, continuous, and persistent anxiety symptoms

(*See also* Generalized Anxiety Disorder; Panic Disorder)

ASSERTIVENESS TRAINING

An alternative therapy that is usually accomplished in groups to help people who tend either to be passive and discount themselves or to be too aggressive. Assertiveness techniques and exercises are designed to teach individuals to ask for what they want and to refuse requests from others without feeling guilty.

ASSESSMENT

Involves nonverbal, verbal, and environmental observations in addition to consideration of the emotive, cognitive, and behavioral aspects of the client. Assessment serves several purposes:

1. Identifying problems
2. Identifying client motivations, strengths, and resources
3. Identifying forces that may hinder the therapeutic plan (forces both internal and external to the client)
4. Setting reasonable goals
5. Determining appropriate intervention strategies
6. Providing continuous evaluation of the process and indicating when the therapeutic plan should be changed

AREAS FOR ASSESSMENT

1. *Physical and intellectual factors*
   a. Presence of physical illness and/or disability
   b. Appearance and energy level
   c. Current and potential levels of intellectual functioning
   d. Perception of personal world
   e. Cause and effect reasoning, ability to focus
2. *Socioeconomic factors*
   a. Level of income, adequacy of subsistence; how this affects lifestyle, sense of adequacy, self-worth
   b. Employment and attitudes about it
   c. Racial, cultural, and ethnic identification; sense of identity and belonging
   d. Religious identification and link to significant value systems, norms, and practices
3. *Personal values and goals*
   a. Presence or absence of congruence between

values and their expression in action; meaning of values to individual

b. Congruence between values and goals and the immediate systems with which client interacts

c. Congruence between values and assessor's values; meaning of this for intervention process

4. *Adaptive functioning and response to present involvement*

a. Manner in which individual presents self to others—grooming, appearance, posture

b. Emotional tone and change or constancy of levels

c. Style of communication (verbal and nonverbal); ability to express appropriate emotion, follow train of thought; factors of dissonance, confusion, uncertainty

d. Symptoms or symptomatic behavior

e. Quality of relationship individual seeks to establish; direction, purposes, and uses of such relationships for individual

f. Perception of self

g. Social roles that are assumed or ascribed; competence in fulfilling these roles

h. Relational behavior
1. Capacity of intimacy
2. Dependence-independence balance
3. Power and control conflicts
4. Exploitiveness
5. Openness

5. *Developmental factors*

a. Role performance equated with life stage

b. Interpretation and uses of previous developmental experiences

c. Methods of coping with past conflicts, tasks, and problems

d. Uniqueness of present problem in life experience

ASTHMA

A disease characterized by labored breathing and wheezing resulting from spasm, secretion, and swelling in the bronchial tree. There are allergic, immunologic, and emotional inputs to asthmatic attacks. The emotional components may lead directly to alterations in bronchus size; they may also affect the allergic and immunologic systems through hypothalamic nuclei in the central nervous system. Because breathing is essential to life itself, there has been much speculation about the emotional and symbolic significance that can become attached to the processes of air exchange.

(*See also* Psychophysiologic Disorder)

AUTISM

Relating to private, individual affects and ideas that are derived from internal drives, hopes, and wishes. Most commonly refers to the private reality of persons labeled schizophrenic as opposed to the shared reality of the external world.

AUTISTIC CHILD

The autistic child is one who from infancy has not engaged in interaction with others.

Assessment

The following characterize the autistic child:

- lack of involvement with others
- lack of verbal communication
- preoccupation with inanimate objects
- ritualistic behavior that preserves routine and sameness

Nursing Intervention

- Meet the child's basic needs to reduce tension and decrease the need for defensive behavior
- Help the child form a relationship with another person (a personal object relationship)
- Help the child develop a sense of self-identity
- Offer the child an opportunity to regress and relive previous developmental stages that were unsuccessfully resolved
- Help the child learn to communicate effectively
- Prevent the child from hurting self or others
- Help the child maintain physical health
- Help the child form relationships with others
- Promote reality testing by the child

AUTONOMIC NERVOUS SYSTEM

That part of the nervous system that controls basic life-sustaining functions such as heart rate, digestion, and breathing; includes the sympathetic nervous system and the parasympathetic nervous system.

Autonomic Nervous System Responses

Organ	Sympathetic Response	Parasympathetic Response
Adrenal medulla	Secretes epinephrine and norepinephrine	None
Heart	Rate increases Force of contraction increases	Rate decreases
Blood vessels to skeletal muscles, heart, brain	Dilate; blood flow increases	Constrict; blood flow decreases

Organ	Sympathetic Response	Parasympathetic Response
Blood vessels to viscera (stomach, intestines, colon)	Constrict; blood flow decreases	Dilate; blood flow increases
Lungs	Air passages dilate	Air passages constrict
Stomach	Inhibits secretion of acid and pepsin	Secretes acid and pepsin
Salivary glands	Inhibits secretion	Secretes saliva
Liver	Releases sugar	None
Colon	Inhibits action	Increases tone
Rectum	Inhibits action	Releases feces
Genitals	Penis ejaculates (males) Blood vessels constrict (females)	Firm erection (males) Blood vessels dilate (females)
Pupils of eyes	Dilate	Constrict
Sweat glands and palms of hands	Secrete sweat	None

B

BAD TRIP
An acute anxiety and panic reaction by a user of psychedelic drugs.

(*See also* Drug Use: General Drug Use Guide for Quick Reference)

BEHAVIOR MODIFICATION
An effort to change "disturbed" or "disordered" behavior through modification techniques. The goal is to remove the symptom. This is done systematically by:

- Identifying and specifying the behavior to be changed, developed, or modified (stopping temper tantrums for example)
- Recording behavior, including frequency, and circumstances
- Determining what conditions maintain the behavior (the child is given candy to stop throwing tantrums)
- Determining how to change these conditions and using reinforcements to decrease unwanted behavior and increase desirable behavior

BENDER-GESTALT TEST
(*See also* Psychologic Tests)

BIOLOGIC THERAPIES
The treatment of emotionally disturbed or incapacitated clients by physiologic means. Also called somatotherapies.

(*See also* Electroconvulsive Therapy; Electrosleep

Therapy; Narcotherapy; Niacin Therapy; Nonconvulsive Electrical Stimulation Therapy; Psychosurgery; Appendix **B,** Psychotropic Drugs; Somatotherapy)

BIPOLAR AFFECTIVE DISORDER (MANIC DEPRESSIVE DISORDER)

Flight of ideas, exalted mood, and pressure of activity during mania; sadness or anxious moodiness and sluggishness of thought and action during depression. A key factor is a history of previous depressive or manic episodes. Clients with bipolar affective disorder are characterized by:

- Normal development and good premorbid adjustment
- Earlier hyperactive behavior and/or an early and critical loss of a significant other and/or a family background of high expectations
- Membership in certain nationality or ethnic groups, such as Scandinavians and Jews
- A family history of bipolar affective disorder (Schizophrenia in the family is less likely.)
- Previous mild mood disturbances.

Nursing Intervention

- Lithium and/or antipsychotic medications
- Hospitalization for clients with severely disturbed behavior to control acute symptoms
- Supportive or relationship therapy to help client understand process of a specific condition and the treatment associated with it
- Family therapy to clear up communication and increase family's understanding of client's problem as a family problem
- Possible long-term maintenance on lithium

(*See also* Depressive Disorder; Manic Behavior)

BLACKY TEST

(See Psychologic Tests)

BLOCKING

The expression of a thought is stopped in midstream, and in a few seconds a new, unrelated thought is expressed.

(See Psychotic Disorders: Form of Thought)

BODY IMAGE

An individual's concept of the shape, size, and mass of his or her body and its parts; the internalized picture that a person has of the physical appearance of his or her body. Body image is closely allied with self-concept or self-image.

BODY IMAGE ALTERATIONS

Change in an individual's concept of his or her body. Loss is the general theme in all body image alterations.

Assessment

- Body characteristics that people have from birth or acquire early in life seem to have less emotional significance for them than those that arise in adolescence or later.
- A defect, handicap, or change in body function that occurs abruptly is far more traumatic than one that develops gradually.
- The location of a disease or injury greatly affects the emotional response to it. Internal diseases are generally less distressing than external diseases that can be seen by the person and others.
- People generally experience a great threat when the face, genitals, or breasts are involved in change.

Nursing Intervention

- Help clients to acknowledge the loss so that they may move from the stage of shock and disbelief into developing awareness.
- Support clients in their move toward the resolution phase of mourning. If necessary, create opportunities for discussing the disability, its meaning to the client, the problem of compensating for the loss, and the reaction of persons with whom the client will come in contact.
- Help family and friends to overcome attitudes of disapproval, repulsion, or rejection by creating opportunities for them to discuss their fears and concerns.
- Refer clients to support groups.

BORDERLINE PERSONALITY DISORDER

(*See* Personality Disorders)

BULIMIA

A disorder characterized by binge eating; it is commonly encountered among adolescent and young adult women. Individuals with bulimia rapidly consume large quantities of high-calorie food, such as ice cream, cake, or candy, over a limited time, such as a couple of hours. These eating binges are commonly followed by severe self-deprecation leading to self-induced vomiting. Between binges, the client may diet or use cathartics and/or diuretics to try to lose weight. Bulimic episodes may occur as part of anorexia nervosa, but not all individuals with bulimia have the disturbances of body image characteristic of anorexia nervosa, and, although weight may fluctuate, clients with bulimia rarely become as emaciated, as do anorexic clients.

(See also Anorexia Nervosa; Psychophysiologic Disorders)

BURNOUT

A condition in which health professionals lose their concern and feeling for the clients they work with and begin to treat them in detached or dehumanized ways. It is an attempt to cope with the intense stress of interpersonal work by distancing.

STRATEGIES TO REDUCE BURNOUT

- Keep staff:client ratios low. Staff members can give more attention to each client and have time to focus on the positive, nonproblem aspects of the client's life.
- Provide for sanctioned breaks, rather than guilt-arousing escapes, from the work situation.
- Provide some relief from prolonged direct client contact (through shorter work shifts or rotating work responsibilities for instance) so that the same staff members are not always working directly with clients.
- Set up formal or informal programs in which staff members can talk about their problems and get advice and support when they need it.
- Encourage staff members to express, analyze, and share their feelings about burning out. This allows them not only to release pentup feelings but also to get constructive feedback from others and perhaps a new perspective as well.
- Encourage staff members to understand their own motivations in pursuing a health career and to recognize their expectations in working with patients.

C

CARDIAC NEUROSIS

Anxiety resulting from intrapsychic or interpersonal conflict creates a symptom constellation totally mimicking structural severe cardiac disease although the electrocardiogram, exercise test, and other laboratory tests give no evidence of organic pathology. This symptom complex can be incapacitating, leading to phobic avoidance responses and gradual, self-imposed isolation.

SYMPTOMS

Palpitations

Tachycardia

Chest pain

Dyspnea

Easy fatigability

Dizziness

Sweating

Irritability

Faintness

Feeling of impending doom

Although few successful treatments are known, behavioral conditioning and psychotropic medications are often used.

CARDIOVASCULAR DISORDERS

High levels of stress are suspected to have deleterious effects on the heart and vascular system, especially if chronic or repeated. The accompanying effects can influence the heart rate, heart rhythm, blood pressure, and so forth.

PREDISPOSING FACTORS

- Family history of heart disease
- Diet high in saturated fats, cholesterol
- High blood levels of cholesterol, triglycerides, sugar, uric acid
- Hypertension, diabetes, hypothyroidism, renal disease, gout
- Low level of physical activity
- Heavy smoking and eating
- High-pressured lifestyle (Type A personality)

(See also Psychophysiologic Disorder)

CATATONIC STATE (Catatonia)
A state characterized by muscular rigidity and immobility, usually associated with schizophrenia.

(See also Schizophrenia/Schizophrenic Disorder)

CATCHMENT AREA
A geographically circumscribed area comprising a city or several rural communities with 75,000 to 200,000 residents. Used to plan and develop mental health and public health services.

CATHARSIS
A basic process in psychotherapy, in which the client freely puts personal feelings, thoughts, daydreams, and interpersonal problems into words. The process usually produces a feeling of relief.

CENTRAL NERVOUS SYSTEM STIMULANTS
This group of drugs includes caffeine, nicotine, cocaine, and amphetamines. These drugs act on the central nervous system to speed up or stimulate functions.

(*See also* Amphetamine; Cocaine; Nicotine)

CEREBRAL VASCULAR DISEASE
Atherosclerosis, hypertension, thrombosis, hemorrhage, and autoimmune and/or collagen vascular disease may all produce varying degrees of altered cerebral functioning. Atherosclerosis presents as progressive impairment of memory, orientation, intellectual efficiency, and judgment, as well as emotional lability in an older person, frequently with a history of hypertension, diabetes, and angina. With thrombosis, hemorrhage, or embolism, dramatic physical changes dominate the clinical picture. Coma or convulsions are more common central nervous system effects than psychosis. A collagen vascular disease such as periarteritis nodosa or systemic lupus erythematosus, on the other hand, more commonly presents with organic psychosis. Such symptoms may respond to the steroids used to treat the overall illness or may require additional use of antipsychotic medication.

(*See also* Organic Brain Syndrome)

CHECKING PERCEPTIONS
A communication skill in which the therapist shares how he or she perceives and hears the client and asks the client to verify these perceptions. Perception checks are used to make sure that one person understands the other.

(*See also* Appendix **C**, Skills that Foster Effective Communication)

CHILD ABUSE

(*See* Family Violence)

CHILD HEALTH ASSESSMENT

PHYSICAL HEALTH

1. Child
   a. *Current*. Child should have had a physical examination recently to identify any physical problems and rule out an organic basis for the presenting problems. Ask for a copy of the physical or a report from the physician or nurse practitioner who performed it. (Obtain permission from the parents before requesting this information from a colleague.)
   b. *History*. Child's health history may also be obtained from the pediatrician if the child has had regular medical care. If not, ask the parents about the usual childhood diseases, any major illnesses, hospitalizations, allergies, and the child's general state of health. Pregnancy and birth data should also be obtained from the parents. Ask questions such as:

   > How was the pregnancy? Any problems?
   >
   > Was the pregnancy planned?
   >
   > How did you feel about it?
   >
   > How was the delivery?
   >
   > Were there any problems with labor or delivery?
   >
   > How much did the baby weigh?
   >
   > Were there any problems after the baby was born?

2. Family
Ask parents about the general state of health of all family members and serious or chronic illnesses (past and present).

FAMILY COMPOSITION

1. *Marital status and age of parents.* Ask whether family is intact. Are there previous marriages? If a single-parent family, does the other parent have contact with the child? How long have parents been married?

2. *Siblings.* Number and age. If it is a blended or restructured family, ask about other parents or siblings.

3. *Socioeconomic class.* Ask parents about place and length of employment. Ask whether residence is rented or owned, and how large it is.

4. *Families of origin.* Determine if maternal and paternal grandparents are alive. If they and other extended family are in area, are they involved with the nuclear family? Try to get some idea of the parents' relationship to their own parents. This can be done through the use of nondirective questions such as:

a. Are you close to your parents now?
b. How was your childhood?
c. What kind of person was your mother?
d. Would you tell me a little about your father?

REFERRAL DATA

1. *Specific information.* Who made the referral and specifically why was it made? For instance, "Eight-year-old Shannon was referred to this clinic by the Fernwood School, where he was brought to the attention of the school psychologist by his teacher, who reports aggressive, acting-out behavior and poor academic performance of 6 months' duration."

Both the presenting problem and the duration of symptoms are important.

2. Subjective perception of the problem
   a. *By parents.* To obtain the parents' perceptions, ask questions such as

   > What do you see as the problem?
   >
   > What are you particularly concerned about?
   >
   > What would you like me to do for your child?
   >
   > How would you like your child to change?
   >
   > What strengths or positive things do you see in your child?

   If the referral was made by someone other than the parents, such as the school, ask if the parents agree with the statements in it and if the child's behavior is different at home.

   b. *By child.* During the play interview, try to get child's perception of the problem by asking questions such as

   > Can you tell me why you're here?
   >
   > Is there anything worrying you?
   >
   > How are things at school? at home?
   >
   > What do you like to do best?
   >
   > Do you have friends at school? at home?

   Frequently the child is quite anxious and will answer, "I don't know" to all questions. It is important to verbalize the problems by saying something like "You've been having trouble at school lately, and your mother brought you here to see if we can figure out how to help."

DEVELOPMENTAL DATA

1. *Major physiologic milestones.* Ask when child sat

up, walked, talked, was toilet trained, could ride a
bicycle.
2. *Psychosocial milestones.* Ask how child responded
to primary caretakers in infancy; to toilet training.
Ask whether child has friends. What things does
child enjoy doing? The nature of these questions
will be determined by the age of the child. For
instance, the nurse wouldn't focus on the absence of
cooperative peer relationships of a 2-year-old, as
this ability does not develop until later.

CURRENT FUNCTIONING

This is assessed by interview and direct observation of
child. An office with play materials is the best setting.
The parents should not be present during this part of
the assessment, so child will feel more free to reveal
conflicts and problems.

1. *Appearance.* This includes child's size, appearance,
and dress. Avoid vague generalities such as
"appropriate dress."
2. *Affect.* Refers to child's feelings or mood. It can be
assessed throughout the interview. Assess both the
various affects displayed and how appropriate they
are to the topic discussed or the play in which child
is engaged. For instance, a smiling and happy affect
would be appropriate if child was describing a
favorite activity; would be inappropriate if child
was discussing failure in school. Take into account
child's possible anxiety, which may influence
affect.
3. *Orientation.* Refers to child's awareness of time,
place, and person. Ask name, address, birthdate,
age and grade of siblings, where the child is now,
and so forth. Keep developmental age in mind: A
child of 6 who does not understand the concept of
time would not necessarily be disoriented since the

concept of time often is not clear until 8 or 9 years.

4. *Perception.* Refers to the ability to receive and interpret sensory information. Throughout the interview evaluate how child uses his or her senses. Once again, developmental age must be considered: Exploring toys with the mouth would be appropriate for an infant but not for a 6-year-old.

5. *Verbalization and play.* These can indicate child's major concerns or preoccupations, child's perception of his or her specific problem (if any), and child's use of fantasy. Some children verbalize freely. This provides information about their social and cultural environment, their ability to relate, their interests, and so on. Other children verbalize little or not at all. Here the primary source of information will be play, which the nurse must interpret.

6. *Fantasy.* Children's fantasies usually reveal their concerns, preoccupations, experiences, and perceptions. By observing their play, the nurse can often assess their fantasies. Another method is to ask children what they would wish for if they could have three things come true. Drawings, especially if child is willing to comment on them, offer another way to identify fantasies.

7. *Self-concept.* Includes both object relations and identifications. Assess how the child relates to the nurse, how the child interacts with the parents, and how the child separates from the parents. Also use information gathered from play, verbalizations, and fantasy. Having the child draw family portraits and self-portraits usually gives further information.

8. *Neuromuscular Skills and Integration.* Throughout the assessment, observe the child's developmental neuromuscular skills and integration. Activities such as throwing a ball, picking up small objects, or grasping a pencil may also be used. Any suspected

deviations from the developmental norm should be medically evaluated.

CHILDHOOD
(See Table 3 on page 52.)

CHILD, SEVERELY DISTURBED
(See Autistic Child)

CHRONICALLY MENTALLY ILL PERSONS
A diverse population of clients characterized by two major disabilities: (1) a limited set of instrumental and problem-solving behaviors that restrict the client in meeting life goals and appear as problems in work, social, and leisure activities, and (2) extreme dependency needs resulting in a reliance on families and institutions. These clients include overlapping populations of those with serious mental disorders, those with disabled and impaired role performance, and those who chronically use psychiatric services (the latter estimated at 1.7–2.4 million in the United States).

Assessment

The chronically mentally ill client has needs and requires resources for:
- Being taken care of
- Social interaction
- Relief of psychiatric symptoms
- Basic life necessities
- Hope

Nursing Intervention

Two programs that have been effective with this group of clients are: (1) Training in Community Living, and
(Continued on page 56)

TABLE 3. NORMAL DEVELOPMENTAL PROGRESSION IN CHILDHOOD

ORAL STAGE	ANAL STAGE	OEDIPAL STAGE	LATENCY STAGE
(Birth to approximately 1 year)	(Approximately 1-3 years)	(Approximately 3-6 years)	(Approximately 6-12 years)
Basic Task	**Basic Task**	**Basic Task**	**Basic Task**
To achieve basic trust versus mistrust	To achieve autonomy versus shame and doubt	To achieve a sense of initiative versus guilt	To achieve a sense of industry versus inferiority
Methods Used:	**Methods Used:**	**Methods Used:**	**Methods Used:**
Oral Exploration. Sucking, biting, spitting, mouthing used to examine environment, express feelings, obtain food	*Exploration.* Continuing to explore, experiment, and manipulate environment (ability to walk allows wider range); exploring own body through masturbation	*Fantasy.* Used for development of initiative through which identity is explored	*Exploration.* Expanding world to neighborhood and school, allows child to try out roles and values in various social and authoritative situations, learning acceptance of responsibility for own behavior, appropriate responses to situations, and acceptance of reasonable res-
Crying and Other Preverbal Vocalizations. Used to communicate with others	*Language.* Used for verbal communication of needs, feelings, and desires	*Exploration.* Expanded mental and locomotor capabilities allow further exploration of self and environment; dimension of planning added to exploration	
Gratification. Obtained			

when biologic needs are met, and infant and caregiver both experience fulfillment

Exploration. Use of eyes, arms, and legs—as well as mouth—to explore environment, making it familiar rather than frightening

Manifestations of Unsuccessful Accomplishment:

Inability to trust, and so to form meaningful relationships with others.

Extreme psychologic dependence

Control. Body used to give or withhold part of self (bowel movement) to control others or to express feelings; important in helping child learn to give, take, and choose (willingness to delay gratification at the request of others can bring increased sense of control and satisfaction; an important step in the socializing process)

Manifestations of Unsuccessful Accomplishment:

Lowered self-esteem and feelings of doubt and shame exhibited by:

Extremely negativistic behavior

Passive-aggressive

Developing Sense of Self. Learning about family and sex roles and how to associate with peers; beginning to observe own actions and thoughts (beginning of adult superego)

Manifestations of Unsuccessful Accomplishment:

Sense of guilt rather than initiative or sense of guilt linked to sense of initiative

Confused sex role

---

trictions and demands

Peer Relationships. Learning cooperation, compromise, and competition

Mastery. Earns recognition by mastering skills and tasks that result in production of things; leads to sense of industry and accomplishment

Manifestations of Unsuccessful Accomplishment:

Feelings of inferiority and inadequacy if child despairs of skills or status among peers

Conflicts in sexual

(Continued)

53

TABLE 3. NORMAL DEVELOPMENTAL PROGRESSION IN CHILDHOOD (Continued)

ORAL STAGE	ANAL STAGE	OEDIPAL STAGE	LATENCY STAGE
Manifestations of Unsuccessful Accomplishment:	**Manifestations of Unsuccessful Accomplishment:**	**Manifestations of Unsuccessful Accomplishment:**	**Manifestations of Unsuccessful Accomplishment:**
Compulsive eating or drinking in attempt to reduce anxiety and satisfy needs for love and security	behavioral patterns Obsessive or compulsive neurosis Sadistic or masochistic tendencies	identification Faulty superego development	identification Continuation of "chum" love and incapacity to direct love toward a member of the opposite sex
Benchmarks in Development:	**Benchmarks in Development:**	**Benchmarks in Development:**	**Benchmarks in Development:**
1 day–1 month. Crawling movements, responds to heat	*1½ years.* Scribbles, knows ten words, can build two-cube tower, has bowel training capability	*3½ years.* Can walk on a line, will take turns, talks to both self and others	*7 years.* Knows days of week, can make simple opposite analogies
1 month. Makes a fist, displays tonic neck reflex, follows object to midline, coos and gurgles	*2 years.* Can build six-cube tower	*4 years.* Can copy an "x", can throw overhand	*8 years.* Can count five digits forward, can define some abstract terms such as "brave" and "nonsense".
	2½ years. Can name six	*4½ years.* Can copy a square	

2 months. Follows object 180°, exhibits social smile, shows suck and grasp reflexes

4 months. Will reach for object

5 months. Can roll over

6-8 months. Sits, crawls, uses raking, grasps

9 months. Can intentionally release objects

10 months. Exhibits pincer grasp

10-14 months. Walks, uses three or four words

body parts, talks in three-word sentences and uses pronouns

3 years. Can match four colors, can copy a circle, can ride a tricycle

5 years. Can copy a triangle, can tie knots in string

6 years. Can tie shoes, can ride two-wheeler, can copy a diamond, can print name, can make single-function similarities

9 years. Knows seasons, rhymes

10 years. Can count four digits backwards, can define more sophisticated abstract terms such as "pity" and "grief"

(2) Alternatives to Hospitalization: residential care through Enabler or foster placements. Both include:

- Assessment
- Daily schedule of activities
- Psychotropic medication
- Strengthening of family and community support systems
- Social activities
- Work time in sheltered employment
- Housing
- Counseling

CIRCUMSTANTIALITY

A disturbance in associative thought processes in which a person digresses into unnecessary details and inappropriate thoughts before communicating the central idea.

CLARIFYING

A communication skill in which the nurse attempts to understand the basic nature of a client's statement by helping to make the meaning clearer.

(See also Appendix C, Skills that Foster Effective Communication)

CLIENT

A consumer of health services. This term is used instead of patient by some mental health professionals.

CLIENT GOVERNMENT GROUPS

Most therapeutic milieus have numerous group activities. One of the commonest is some form of client government. Client governments take many forms, but in most cases staff and clients meet together once or twice a week to discuss and resolve day-to-day issues on the ward. Key principles in client government are:

- Client government should ideally make and enforce most of the ward rules.
- Client government should organize and execute most of the routine ward tasks.
- No staff member should attempt to solve a problem if it can be delegated to the client government.

Client government offers:

- A way of making life in a mental hospital resemble life in the external community
- A way of controlling deviant behavior with group pressure
- Group support for very disturbed clients
- A way of increasing recreational activities
- An opportunity for clients to understand administrative policy and help formulate it
- A way of increasing clients' self-esteem
- An opportunity for clients to express annoyances and resentments
- A channel of communication between clients and staff members providing ways of improving morale and of uncovering and working out tensions

CLINICAL PSYCHOLOGIST

A psychologist specially educated and trained in the area of mental health. Certification is at the doctoral level after the candidate has completed a one-year internship at an approved facility. Clinical psychologists perform psychotherapy, plan and implement programs of behavior modification, and select, administer, and interpret psychologic tests.

COCAINE

Acts as a topical anesthetic. Among users it is usually sniffed or snorted rather than injected intravenously.

If taken in sufficient quantity, it induces euphoric excitement and hallucinatory experiences. Despite its comparatively high cost in the street market, its use is increasing. As with amphetamines and other stimulants, users experience depression when they stop using it. Heavy use of this stimulant can cause a particular kind of drug-induced psychosis called *cocaine bugs*, in which sufferers feel that bugs are crawling under their skin.

(*See also* Substance Use Disorders)

COGNITIVE
Related to the mental processes of thought, memory, comprehension, and reasoning.

(*See also* Mental Status Examination)

COHESIVENESS
A sense of belonging; the result of all the forces acting on members to remain in a group.

COLIC
Involves crying that usually is confined to one part of the day and starts after a feeding.

It commonly begins in the first to third month and may be caused by sharp intestinal pains produced by gas, possibly due to periodic tension in the infant's immature nervous system.

Intervention consists of reassuring the parents and giving them information about the condition. Hot water bottles, rocking, rubbing the back, or a pacifier may soothe the infant.

COMMITMENT
The legal process by which a person is confined to a mental hospital. It may be voluntary or involuntary.

(*See also* Legal Aspects)

COMMUNICATION

An ongoing, dynamic, and ever-changing series of events in which one event influences all the others. Responding with meaning is the essence of effective communication. Meaning must be mutually negotiated between persons.

STRATEGIES FOR COMMUNICATING WITH CLIENTS FROM DIFFERENT CULTURES

1. If you don't speak the language of your client try:
   a. Enlisting aid of a family member or friend of the client
   b. Seeking out a bilingual staff member in the setting
   c. Asking another client to translate
   d. Using other agencies as resources
2. Select carefully the words you use, avoiding buzz words and jargon. Speak clearly, pacing yourself to be neither too fast nor too slow.
3. Select with care the gestures you use, using nonverbal behavior to underscore your words and actions.
4. Listen to your client's words and watch your client's gestures carefully. Do your best to understand and validate the meaning they have for you.

(*See* Appendix **C,** Skills that Foster Effective Communication)

COMMUNITY MENTAL HEALTH

A system for the delivery of mental health services based on a shift from institutional to community-based care in which primary, secondary, and tertiary prevention are emphasized.

COMMUNITY MENTAL HEALTH CENTER

Center for applying community mental health concepts. Centers include inpatient (24-hour) facilities, partial hospitalization facilities (such as day, night, and weekend hospitals), outpatient departments, emergency services, consultation services, and education programs.

COMPULSION

An uncontrollable, persistent urge to perform certain acts or behaviors to relieve an otherwise unbearable tension. There are two kinds of compulsive acts: (1) those that give expression to the primary impulses, and (2) those that are attempts to undo or control these impulses. Most compulsive acts are attempts to control or modify obsessions, either because of fear of the consequences or fear of the inability to control the primary impulse.

Typical compulsive acts are endless handwashing, checking and rechecking doors to see if they have been locked, and elaborate dressing and undressing rituals. Such defensive acts are used to contain, neutralize, or ward off anxiety related to the primary impulse.

(*See also* Obsession; Compulsive Personality Disorder)

COMPULSIVE PERSONALITY DISORDER

An excessive conformity and conscientiousness. Persons with this disorder are excessively meticulous and perfectionistic.

Assessment

Among the features generally associated with compulsive life styles are rigidity, the distortion of the experience of autonomy, and the loss of consensual reality. Extremely maladaptive forms involve elaborate and at times health-threatening compulsive rituals. Other characteristics include:

1. Inability to receive a casual or immediate impression
2. Concentration on insignificant details
3. Selective inattention to any new idea or external influence (because of rigid cognitive model)
4. Insensitivity to the emotional tone of social situations
5. Sense of deliberateness; lack of spontaneity
6. Activity that seems pressed or motivated by something beyond the client's own interest
7. Lack of enthusiasm for pursued activities
8. Difficulty with decision making and free choice
9. Attempt to reach a solution by calling on some rule or external requirement
10. In severe cases, worries bordering on the delusional
11. Lack of personal convictions
12. Inability to see things in their real proportions

Nursing Intervention

1. Coping with the compulsive behavior. Interference with rituals must be carefully weighed and timed to match the client's progress in psychotherapy.
2. Attempting to develop an affirming, dependable relationship with clients before suggesting that they change their behavior patterns.
3. Balancing the value of intervening in behavior that protects clients from mental anguish against the need to prevent physical deterioration caused by the behavior.
4. Dealing with the client's communication problem. Pedantic striving for accuracy produces greater vagueness and confusion.
5. Working with the client's dependency conflict. The dependence-independence conflict is usually encountered in one form or another.

6. Discovering the source of the original anxiety that caused the client's obsessive-compulsive behavior.

(*See also* Personality Disorders)

CONCRETE THINKING
A primitive type of thinking that assumes that ideas have a literal, superficial meaning. It is characteristic of children, retarded individuals, and schizophrenics.

CONDITIONING
Learning that occurs through reinforcement in which behaviors are rewarded and thus persist or are punished and thus stopped.

(*See* Behavior Modification)

CONDUCT DISORDERS (behavior problems)
A means by which latency-stage children express their conflicts. This includes nonproductive behavior that is repeated despite threats, punishments, or rational arguments. The child is expressing and communicating conflicts through behavior, rather than verbally. Conduct disorders may be aggressive (in which the basic rights of others are violated) or nonaggressive.

Treatment involves counseling or therapy for the child by a psychiatric nurse or other mental health worker allowing the child to resolve the basic conflict thus making the problem behavior unnecessary.

CONFLICT
A state in which opposing desires, feelings, or goals coexist. Conflict increases tension and provides energy, and thus it is a crucial factor in behavior. When persons cannot use the energy to resolve the conflict, they are often left with a stalemate. To diminish the

anxiety associated with the conflict they may make maladaptive responses: hesitation, blocking, fatigue, vacillation, tension, and/or withdrawal. Most likely to cause anxiety are conflicts that involve: social relations with significant people, ethical standards, meeting unconscious needs, or problems of everyday family living.

A conflict proceeds as follows:

1. The person holds two goals simultaneously.
2. The person moves in relation to both of the goals, using approach-avoidance movements, or avoidance-avoidance movements.
3. The person shows hesitation, vacillation, blocking, or fatigue.
4. Resolution occurs either temporarily or permanently.

CONFRONTATION

Deliberate invitation to another to examine some aspect of personal behavior in which there is a discrepancy between what the person says and what he or she does. Confrontation requires careful attention to nonverbal communication and the discrepancies between nonverbal and verbal messages.

Confrontations may be informational or interpretive, and they may be directed toward both the resources and the limitations of the client. An informational confrontation describes the visible behavior of another person; an interpretive confrontation expresses thoughts and feelings about another's behavior and includes drawing inferences about the meaning of that behavior.

(See also Appendix C, Skills That Foster Effective Communication)

CONFUSION

Disordered, jumbled thinking. It is the most common emotional, behavioral, and cognitive reaction to stressors in old age.

A mild confusional tendency and disturbed behavior may simply indicate sensory impairment, a lack of structure, insufficient environmental cues (clocks, calendars), or lack of attention to such cues. A deprived, boring environment will often induce a state of confusion. Preoccupation with fears, losses, or threats to security and independence may also appear as confusion. More pronounced confusional states leading to disruptive behaviors often follow translocation, environmental overload, and acute grief.

The most devastating confusional states, including severe disorientation, occur with severe overtaxing of physiologic homeostatic mechanisms by injuries, toxic conditions, metabolic deficiencies, impaired cerebral metabolism (enzymatic or circulatory), and disease processes. In other words, anything that taxes the limits of homeostatic resilience may result in temporary disintegrative patterns, confusion, and disorientation.

ORIENTATION GUIDELINES FOR WORKING WITH CONFUSED CLIENTS

- Add as many visual cues to the setting as you can. When vision is impaired, consistent auditory input is essential. Check hearing aids and eyeglasses for effective function.
- Make the environment as predictable as possible by anticipatory planning and a safe, routine, printed schedule. When changes must be made, introduce them slowly and rehearse expected performance with the individual involved.
- Arrange for a thorough physical and neurologic

examination to rule out an organic basis for confusion. Remember, however, that too many intrusive or diagnostic procedures in a short time will increase confusion.

- Assess the stresses experienced recently and within the last 2 years.
- If sensory deprivation or lack of stimulation is the problem, add color, texture, flavor, and noncompetitive activity to the daily schedule. If an overload of new expectations and adaptations has occurred, increase environmental stability, reduce expectations, and promote rest and continuity of supportive personnel.
- When confusion is extensive and organically based, reduce expectations to those that can be accomplished and give consistent, immediate praise for any degree of success. This must be done by all personnel, and long-term, consistent efforts are essential.
- Establish a relationship that conveys the value of the client regardless of functional capacity.
- Develop a solid peer support system for yourself. Those who understand the disappointments and struggles of nursing are in the best position to listen to each other. Sharing feelings, anger, exasperation, and humor help the nurse continue in a very difficult task.

(*See also* Aged Persons)

CONTRACT

A plan of action and goals mutually negotiated between client and mental health professional. Can be compared to the *nursing care plan*, but the contract focuses more on client input and therapist/staff accountability.

CONVERSION REACTION

Pre-DSM-III term for a disturbed personal coping pattern in which an anxiety-provoking impulse is converted into somatic symptoms.

(*See also* Somatoform Disorder)

COPING MECHANISMS

An adaptive method or capacity developed by a person to deal with or overcome a psychologic or social problem.

COUNTERTRANSFERENCE

Sigmund Freud's term for irrational attitudes taken by an analyst toward a patient. It may create problems in psychotherapeutic work. The therapist needs to become aware of countertransference and seek consistent supervision to intervene when it occurs.

COUPLES THERAPY

An extension of the more traditional marital therapy to the therapy of interactional dyads when difficulties between the partners are specific to their relationship.

CRISIS

A situation in which customary problem-solving or decision-making methods are no longer adequate; a state of psychological disequilibrium. A crisis may be a turning point in a person's life. A crisis is self-limiting: It lasts a few days to a few weeks and will eventually run its course with or without intervention. However, the person who experiences a crisis alone is more vulnerable to unsuccessful negotiation than the person who works through a crisis with help.

TYPES OF CRISES

TYPE	DEFINITION	EXAMPLES
Developmental	Crisis that occurs in response to stresses common to all persons in periods of human maturation and transition	Birth, early childhood, preschool, puberty, adolescence, young adulthood, late adulthood, adulthood, old age
Situational	Crisis that occurs in response to stressful or traumatic external events	
Anticipated	Expected event for which some preparation is possible	Beginning nursery school, birth of sibling, divorce of parents, dating, job promotion
Unanticipated	Unexpected and usually chance event that involved person has not predicted and is unprepared to meet	Death of significant person before old age, imprisonment, hospitalization for acute illness
Victim	Traumatic event involving physically aggressive and forced act	War, rape, civil riot, murder, assault, incest

TYPE	DEFINITION	EXAMPLES
	by another per- son or by environment	

(*See also* Crisis Counseling; Crisis Intervention)

CRISIS COUNSELING

Crisis counseling is brief (five to six sessions) and issue-oriented. The counsellor makes an assessment and helps the client explore assessment issues.

Hoff suggests that healthy crisis coping can be achieved if the nurses will*:

- Listen actively and with concern
- Encourage open expression of feelings
- Help client gain an understanding of crisis
- Help client gradually accept reality
- Help client explore new ways of coping with problems
- Link client to a social network
- Engage in decision counseling or problem solving with the client
- Reinforce newly learned coping devices
- Followup client after resolution of crisis

CRISIS INTERVENTION

A therapeutic strategy which views people as capable of personal growth and able to control their own lives.

This process is aimed at re-establishing the client's functioning at a level equal to or better than the precrisis level. Effective planning for crisis resolution must be:

- Based on careful assessment

*Hoff, L.A. 1984. *People in Crisis: Understanding and Helping,* 2nd ed. Menlo Park, Calif.: Addison-Wesley Publishing Co., p. 120.

- Developed in active collaboration with the person in crisis and the significant others in that person's life
- Focused on immediate, concrete, contributing problems
- Based on an understanding of human dependence needs
- Appropriate to the crisis-ridden person's level of thinking, feeling, and behaving
- Consistent with the person's lifestyle and culture
- Time limited, concrete, and realistic
- Mutually negotiated and renegotiated
- Organized to provide for followup

(*See also* Lethality Assessment; Suicide)

CUSHING'S DISEASE
An excess of adrenal cortical hormones such as that associated with glandular tumor, hyperplasia, or iatrogenic administration of cortisone-like drugs.

Assessment

Clients may exhibit euphoria, heightened sense of well-being, or mania, with or without psychosis. Physically clients characteristically have a round face, thick neck, obese trunk, and accumulated fat on shoulders, arms, and legs. Hirsutism; thin, easily bruised skin; and purple striae on the thighs and abdomen are common. Diagnosis is made by measuring levels of steroids excreted in the urine, which are elevated when the disease is present.

Treatment

Depending on the cause, treatment may be surgical removal or stopping the administration of exogenous agents.

(*See also* Endocrine Disorders; Organic Brain Syndrome)

CYCLOTHYMIC DISORDER

An affective disorder characterized by recurring episodes of high and low moods.

(*See also* Bipolar Affective Disorder)

D

DECOMPENSATION
Disorganization of a previously stable emotional adjustment or defensive system.

DEFENSE MECHANISMS
Operations outside of a person's awareness that the ego calls into play to protect against anxiety; the psychoanalytic term for coping mechanisms (also called mental mechanisms). They protect the self by enabling denial or distortion of a stressful event or by restricting awareness and reducing the sense of emotional involvement. They can also interfere with rational decision making. People who use defense mechanisms are excluding some information about the situation they are in and denying their own feelings about it.

Specific Defense Mechanisms

NAME	DEFINITION	EXAMPLE
Repression	Unacceptable feelings are unconsciously kept out of awareness	A man is jealous of a good friend's success but unaware of his feelings.
Suppression	Unacceptable feelings and thoughts are consciously kept out of awareness	A student taking an examination is upset about an argument with her boyfriend but puts it out of her mind so she

NAME	DEFINITION	EXAMPLE
		can finish the test.
Identification	Unconscious assumption of similarity between oneself and another	After hospitalization for minor surgery a girl decides to be a nurse.
Introjection	Acceptance of another's values and opinions as one's own	A woman who prefers a simple life style assumes the materialistic, prestige-oriented values of her husband.
Projection	One's own unacceptable feelings and thoughts are attributed to others	A man who is quite critical of others thinks that people are joking about his appearance.
Denial	Blocking out painful or anxiety-inducing events or feelings	A boss tells an employee he may have to fire him; on the way home the employee shops for a new car.
Fantasy	Symbolic satisfaction of wishes through	A student struggling through gradu-

NAME	DEFINITION	EXAMPLE
	nonrational thought	ate school thinks about a prestigious, high-paying job he wants.
Rationalization	Falsification of experience through the construction of logical or socially approved explanations of behavior	A man cheats on his income tax return and tells himself it's all right because everyone does it.
Reaction formation	Unacceptable feelings disguised by repression of the real feeling and by reinforcement of the opposite feeling	A woman who dislikes her mother-in-law is always very nice to her.
Displacement	Discharging of pentup feelings on persons less dangerous than those who initially aroused the emotion	A student who has received a low grade on a term paper blows up at his girlfriend when she asks about his grade.
Intellectualization	Separating an emotion from	A man learns from his doctor

NAME	DEFINITION	EXAMPLE
	an idea or thought because the emotional reaction is too painful to be acknowledged	that he has cancer; he studies the physiology and and treatment of cancer without experiencing any emotion.

DEINSTITUTIONALIZATION

The shift of care and funding arrangements for the chronically and severely mentally ill from single-purpose, custodial state hospitals to multipurpose services based near clients' families and communities.

DÉJÀ VU

An illusion of visual recognition in which a new situation is incorrectly regarded as a repetition of a previous experience. This phenomenon occurs occasionally in everyone's life, but the schizophrenic is likely to report it with great frequency.

DELIRIUM

Confusion in thinking often accompanied by fear. It stems from an acute organic reaction and is characterized by restlessness, confusion, disorientation, bewilderment, agitation, and affective lability.

(*See also* Confusion)

DELIRIUM TREMENS

An acute psychotic state usually occurring after a prolonged and copious intake of alcohol.

(*See also* Alcohol/Alcoholic/Alcoholism)

DELUSION

An important personal belief that is almost certainly not true and is resistant to modification.

COMMON DELUSIONS

- *Delusion of alien control.* Feelings of being controlled or guided by external forces. Ask the client, "Do you ever feel your thoughts or actions are under outside influences or control? Are you able to influence others, to read their minds, or to put thoughts in their minds?"

- *Delusion of being controlled.* Belief that individual's feelings, impulses, thoughts, or actions are not his or her own but are imposed from some external source.

- *Bizarre delusion.* Content of delusion is so absurd that there is no possible way it could be based on fact.

- *Delusion of grandeur.* Belief that individual has a special relationship to the world, for example, that he or she is a prominent person, living or dead, or is related to such a person.

- *Delusion of persecution.* Belief that individual is harassed, in danger, under investigation, and/or at the mercy of some powerful force.

- *Delusion of reference.* Belief that certain events, situations, or interactions are directly related to oneself.

- *Nihilistic delusion.* More or less complete denial of reality and existence; client states that nothing exists, or everything is lost.

- *Delusion of self-depreciation.* Feelings of unworthiness, sinfulness, ugliness, or emitting obnoxious odors. Often seen in connection with severe depressions.

- *Somatic Delusions.* Belief that individual's body is

changing or responding in some unusual way. He or
she may be unaware of ordinary sensations such as
hunger or thirst.

(*See also* Bipolar Affective Disorder; Mental Status
Examination; Schizophrenia)

DEMENTIA

Chronic organic mental syndrome. Onset may be
either acute or insidious, without clouding of level of
consciousness. Recent memory becomes impaired
first; personality change is prominent and brain damage is evident.

DENIAL

A defense mechanism, or coping mechanism, by which
the mind refuses to acknowledge a thought, feeling,
wish, need, or reality factor. The reality of a situation
is either completely disregarded or is transformed so
that it is no longer threatening.

In some cases, denial is the best solution for the
client, and it should be supported. However, when
denial is harmful to the client, the motivation for the
client's behavior should be assessed. Once the particular protective function the denial is serving has been
discovered, the nurse can focus attention on helping
the client meet these needs in a way that is not self-
destructive.

(*See also* Defense Mechanisms)

DEPENDENT PERSONALITY DISORDER

Disruptive life styles having the common characteristic of fearfulness; in DSM III, it includes avoidant,
dependent, and passive-aggressive personalities:

- *Avoidant personality.* These clients are hypersensi-
  tive to potential rejection, yet experience a strong
  need for acceptance and affection.

- *Dependent personality.* These clients passively allow others to assume responsibility for major areas of their lives because of low self-esteem and lack of self-confidence.
- *Passive-Aggressive Personality.* These clients appear dependent and lack self-confidence, but their most consistent characteristic is resistance to demands for occupational and social performance expressed indirectly through such maneuvers as procrastination, dawdling, stubbornness, inefficiency, and forgetfulness. These behaviors persist even under circumstances in which more assertive and effective patterns are possible.

Nursing Intervention

- Anticipate clients' needs before they demand attention
- Set realistic limits about what can and cannot be done for clients
- Help clients manage anxiety that occurs when others do not spontaneously meet their needs
- Teach clients to express their ideas and feelings assertively
- Support clients who are gradually making more of their own decisions

(*See also* Personality Disorders)

DEPERSONALIZATION

A dissociative phenomenon, characterized by feelings of strangeness or unreality of the self or the environment. It is not uncommon among clients whose functioning is disintegrative.

DEPERSONALIZATION DISORDER

The essential feature is one or more episodes of alteration in the perception or experience of the self so that the usual sense of personal reality is temporarily lost or changed with subsequent social or occupational impairment.

(*See also* Dissociative Disorders)

DEPRESSIVE DISORDER

Usually originates with an experience of loss. Common features of depressive disorders are loss of ambition, boredom, and numerous physical complaints. The latter include fatigue, loss of appetite (anorexia), sleep disturbances (including both excessive sleeping and insomnia), and loss of libido. People who rely on depressive reactions as a coping strategy have few inner resources to combat threats to their self-esteem and become extremely despondent.

Assessment

- Alteration in feeling toward sadness, loneliness, and apathy
- Vegetative physical changes
- Alteration in activity level toward either retardation or agitation
- Lowered self-esteem associated with self-reproaches and blame
- History (usually recent) of experienced loss

CLINICAL PICTURE OF DEPRESSION

1. Muscles of the face droop, giving a glum, dispirited appearance.
2. Eyeballs may be sunken because of weight loss.
3. When seated, client assumes a slumped position; when walking, gait is slow and dragging.
4. Crying is frequent.
5. Sleep problems are common.
6. Disinterest in personal hygiene is evident; clients appear dirty and disheveled.

7. Retardation of various systems (including gastrointestinal tract with resultant constipation) may occur.
8. Harsh self-criticism is frequent.
9. Feelings of worthlessness are evident.
10. Passive, clinging, beseechingly dependent behavior may be apparent.

Factors related to the development of depression include:

1. Biologic
   a. Possible genetic influence
   b. Hormonal influence (drop in estrogen and progesterone)
   c. Biochemical activities of monoamine oxidase and catecholamines (high levels)
2. Psychologic
   a. Dependency
   b. Low self-esteem
   c. Powerlessness
   d. Ambivalence
   e. Guilt
3. Cognitive
   a. Narrow, negative perspective of self, world, and future
   b. Conclusions drawn on inadequate or contradictory evidence
   c. Overgeneralizations from one instance
   d. Focus on single detail rather than on whole
   e. Distortion of long-range consequences, hence bad judgment
4. Sociocultural
   a. Status of minority groups
   b. Status of women in male-oriented professional and business culture
   c. Role loss (as loss of head of household role)

d. Being the object of cultural stereotyping (for instance, blacks, aged, Jews)

Table 4 differentiates between major depressive episode, bipolar affective disorder, and dysthymic disorder.

DEPRESSION ALGORITHM

An algorithm such as the one provided in the following chart offers a set of step-by-step instructions for collecting data about a depressed client. Nursing intervention for depressed clients is then geared toward helping them meet their needs for safety, hygiene, rest, activity, nutrition, elimination, self-esteem, and affiliation.

ALGORITHM FOR DEPRESSION*

For use when client indicates problem related to depressed mood, feelings of guilt or shame, or when client exhibits agitation or lethargy not immediately attributable to organic cause

Depressed Mood (Guilt, Agitation, Lethargy)

↓	↓
Identifies sources of depressed state	After describes problem, explore for client's ideas about possible precipitating events
↓	↓
Do possible sources include:	Client cannot identify any possible precipitants. This may indicate:
1. Recent loss or threat	

(Continued on page 82.)

*Reprinted with permission from *Journal of Psychiatric Treatment and Evaluation*, Marcia Orsolits and Murray Morphy. "A Depression Algorithm for Psychiatric Emergencies" (in press), Pergamon Press, Ltd.

80

TABLE 4. DEPRESSION AND RELATED DISORDERS

CRITERIA	MAJOR DEPRESSIVE EPISODE	BIPOLAR DISORDER	DYSTHYMIC DISORDER
Intensity	Depressive symptoms prominent	Depressive symptoms prominent	Depressive symptoms mild
Ego impairment	May have psychotic features	May have psychotic features	No psychotic features
Pattern	No history of manic episode	Has had manic episode	Alternating depressed and hypomaniac periods over 2-year period

of loss (spouse, child, job, income)

Yes_____ No_____

2. Recent illness or recent exacerbation of chronic illness

Yes_____ No_____

↓

1. Endogenous depression or
2. Lack of insight
Both possibilities indicate greater risk to client. Move on to next step now, but use this factor in final evaluation of severity of depression.

Total_____

Ask Client to Confirm or Deny the Following: Yes/No

1. Feeling sad, blue   Yes____ No____
↓
2. Crying spells   Yes____ No____
↓
3. Exaggerated symptoms in morning   Yes____ No____
↓
4. Change in sleeping patterns   Yes____ No____
↓
5. Change in appetite   Yes____ No____
↓
6. Weight loss in past 6 months   Yes____ No____
↓
7. Decreased libido   Yes____ No____
↓
8. G.I. changes (constipation, etc.)   Yes____ No____

↓

9. C.V. changes (tachycardia, etc.)　　　Yes____ No____

↓

10. Unexplained fatigue　　　Yes____ No____

↓

11. Mental confusion　　　Yes____ No____

↓

12. Agitation　　　Yes____ No____

↓

13. Psychomotor retardation　　　Yes____ No____

↓

14. Sense of life being "empty"　　　Yes____ No____

↓

15. Sense of hopelessness　　　Yes____ No____

↓

16. Indecisiveness　　　Yes____ No____

↓

17. Irritability　　　Yes____ No____

↓

18. Sense of dissatisfaction with life　　　Yes____ No____

↓

19. Sense of dissatisfacton with self　　　Yes____ No____

↓

20. Suicidal rumination　　　Yes____ No____

Total____

Client communicates presence
of suicidal thoughts

Client denies any suicidal
thought or intent

Does client feel hopeless
and/or helpless   Yes____ No____

Does client have specific
suicide plan   Yes____ No____

Is plan feasible and lethal   Yes____ No____

Does client abuse alcohol
and/or drugs   Yes____ No____

Is client living alone   Yes____ No____

Does client have close friends
or family readily available   Yes____ No____

Is client over 45, male,
unemployed or retired   Yes____ No____

Total____

Total Yes ____ + ____ + ____ = ____

In Your Judgment Does the Client Have:

Organic brain syndrome   Yes____ No____

Serious financial pressure   Yes____ No____

Hallucinations/delusions   Yes____ No____

↓

History of past suicidal attempt(s)   Yes____ No____

↓

History of poor response to past treatment   Yes____ No____

↓

Poor ability to use available resources   Yes____ No____

Total____

Total Yes _____ + Total Yes _____ = _____ Final Score

Admit to psychiatric unit   5. _____
Refer to:
    Day hospital   4. _____
    Crisis intervention   3. _____
    Outpatient clinic   2. _____
    Home (no treatment)   1. _____

↓   ↑

To M.D.   (Level II or III)
Confirmation   1. _____
Medical evaluation   2. _____

Algorithm Scoring   Add the number of "Yes" responses in each subsection to provide a final score. Scoring has been included in the algorithm's construction from the outset in order to facilitate future analysis of data. Correlations of disposition decisions, and possibly other outcome measures, with these subtotal and total scores can be completed.

Nursing Intervention

1. *Safety.* Severely depressed clients may die of starvation or suicide. They may become so racked with self-doubt and sadness that they become immobilized and stuporous. In these cases, the nurse will need to intervene on the client's behalf. The nurse may have to plan actions that will substitute temporarily for the patient's own protective devices.

2. *Hygiene.* Depressed clients might be unkempt in appearance and have poor hygiene thus risking invasion by pathogens and infection. This also perpetuates the client's low self-esteem. It may be necessary for the nurse to groom depressed clients who are unable to do it for themselves.

3. *Rest and activity.* Fatigue and sleeping disturbances reinforce depression. Sometimes activity (including working at their usual occupation) will help clients increase their self-esteem and also distract them from morbid ruminations. Redirecting the client's attention from the past to the future can help them develop new activities and goals.

4. *Nutrition and elimination.* Depressed clients are subject to malnutrition and serious changes in normal bowel activity. Some ways to minimize these problems are to:

   a. Encourage client to engage in physical activity
   b. Modify client's food intake (increasing fiber for instance)
   c. Monitor client's output for evidence of serious and prolonged constipation

   A consistent, firm approach is often necessary in encouraging clients to follow the suggested treatment regimen.

5. *Self-esteem and affiliation.* Observe the following guidelines:

   Make therapeutic use of self in the form of empathic presence and listening.

Establish a nurse-client relationship that conveys respect, both verbally and nonverbally, for dignity of client. This may be done by keeping promises, following agreements about time structure, and avoiding false reassurances.

Provide an organized, well-planned schedule to help the client fend off the decline to a vegetative state.

Build new communication patterns in which the depressed client can learn to express negative feelings openly instead of turning them inward.

Observe precautions against suicide.

DESENSITIZATION
A process in which a person is exposed serially to a predetermined list of anxiety-provoking situations graded in a hierarchy from the least to the most frightening, with the goal of reducing the anxiety these situations cause.

(*See* Behavior Modification)

DETACHED CONCERN
The ability to distance oneself to help others. It is an essential quality in avoiding burnout, in using appropriate assertiveness when collaborating with colleagues, and in maintaining empathic abilities in highly stressful situations.

(*See* Burnout)

DETACHMENT
Behavioral pattern characterized by generalized aloofness in interpersonal contact. Detachment, as a form of resistance, can retard relationship work and discourage the practitioner. Manifestations of detachment include intellectualization, denial, and superficiality.

Nursing Intervention

- Establish awareness of process of detachment—that is, what client does to remain aloof in interpersonal contact. (Focuses on dysfunctional behavioral pattern and encourages self-awareness)
- Encourage client assessment of how this serves client, including delineation of any self-defeating aspects. (Encourages client to evaluate behavioral pattern to determine which parts are self-defeating and/or thwart gratification of basic needs)
- Explore any fears and fantasies inhibiting emotional expression. (Links thought processes to emotive expression)
- Actively emphasize emotive content. (Interrupts dysfunctional behavioral pattern)

DEVELOPMENTAL STAGES

A series of normative conflicts or specific psychosocial tasks with which every person must deal. Developmental stages are a kind of timetable for personality development specifying the desirable rate of growth or accomplishment and favoring certain aspects of development at the expense of others.

DEVIANCE

Behavior characterized by marked differences in actions, morals, and attitudes from the usual social standards.

DEXAMETHASONE SUPPRESSION TEST (DST)

A diagnostic tool (also called a biologic marker) useful in diagnosing depressive illness and predicting which endogenously depressed patients will respond favorably to tricyclic antidepressant medications that inhibit blood levels of the hormone cortisol. Research indicates that 50% of endogenously depressed clients exhibit an activation of the limbic-hypothalamic-pituitary-adrenal (LHPA) axis and fail to supress plasma cortisol levels on the day following the DST. Abnormal DSTs also occur with Cushing's syndrome, other primary endocrine illnesses, cancer with ectopic adrenocorticotropic hormone production, renovascular hypertension, chronic renal failure, alcohol abstinence syndrome, protein-caloric malnutrition, anorexia nervosa, and obesity.

Procedure

After blood sampling for cortisol, clients usually receive a 1 mg pill (0.5 mg and 2 mg have also been used) of the synthetic steroid dexamethasone. They are instructed to swallow it at 11 PM and to refrain from taking any other drugs including alcohol. The following day a teaspoon of blood is drawn at 4 PM, and the level of cortisol is measured. Variations in the number of blood-sampling points (as many as three on each day) have also been used.

Interpretation

It is possible to attribute the lack of cortisol suppression to (a) hypersecretion of hormones, (b) phase-shifted secretion of hormones altering the critical time of glandular responsiveness, or (c) some other alteration in the LHPA axis that regulates hormonal secretion.

DISASTER RESPONSE

Three overlapping stages have been identified:

1. *Impact.* Stimulated by the catastrophe, victims recognize what is happening to them and are concerned mainly with the present. During this acute phase, victim's major concern may be staying alive.
2. *Recoil.* Initial stress of disaster has passed, and

victims no longer find themselves in immediate danger. Behavior of victims is usually dependent; they want to be taken care of. Weeping is common as survivors begin to realize all that has happened to them.

3. *Post-trauma period.* Grief is predominant response as victims mourn the losses in their lives. Disturbed and disintegrated responses may occur.

Nursing Intervention

Hoff* suggests that disaster victims need an opportunity to (a) Talk out the experience and express their feelings of fear, panic, loss, and grief; (b) become fully aware and accepting of what has happened to them; and (c) resume concrete activity and reconstruct their lives with the social, physical, and emotional resources available. The nurse should thus:

1. Listen with concern and sympathy and ease the way for victims to tell their tragic story, weep, express feelings of anger, loss, frustration, and despair.
2. Help victims accept in small doses the tragic reality of what has happened. This means staying with them during initial stages of shock and denial. It also may mean accompanying them back to the scene of the tragedy and being available for support when they are faced with the full impact of their loss.
3. Assist them to make contact with relatives, friends, and other resources needed to begin the process of social and physical reconstruction. This could mean making telephone calls to locate relatives, accompanying someone to apply for financial aid, giving

*Hoff, L.A. 1984. *People in Crisis: Understanding and Helping,* 2nd ed. Menlo Park, Calif.: Addison-Wesley Publishing Co., p. 289.

information about social and mental health agencies for followup services.

(*See also* Crisis; Post-Traumatic Stress Disorder)

DISORIENTATION
Impairment in the understanding of temporal, spatial, or personal relationships. Lack of awareness of the correct time, place, or person.

DISPLACEMENT
A defense or coping mechanism in which a person discharges pentup feelings on persons less threatening than those who initially aroused the emotion. In some cases, anger aroused by another person may be turned inward on the self. When this happens, the individual will experience exaggerated self-accusations and guilt.

(*See also* Defense Mechanisms)

DISSOCIATION
A coping mechanism that protects the self from a threatening awareness of uncomfortable feelings by denying their existence in awareness. People who express dissociated feelings or qualities do not "notice" what they are doing. This limitation of awareness is maintained because the person experiences anxiety whenever permissible levels for the self are trespassed.

(*See also* Defense Mechanisms)

DISSOCIATIVE DISORDERS
Dissociative coping patterns are somewhat uncommon and often bizarre defensive reactions to stress. There are five types of dissociative reactions:

1. Sleepwalking
2. Amnesia
3. Fugue
4. Multiple personality
5. Depersonalization disorder

These reactions are complex and are usually difficult to distinguish from one another. The common characteristic is that a cluster of recent, related mental events is beyond the client's power of recall but can return spontaneously to conscious awareness. Depersonalization disorder is included because in it the client's feeling of personal reality, an important component of identity, is lost.

A nursing care plan for a client with dissociative coping patterns would include:

- *Physical Assessment.* A meticulous assessment should be made of the client's physical condition to rule out organic causes for the dissociative disorder, such as brain tumor. (*See* Physiologic and Neurologic Assessment.) Nurses' observations of the descriptive character, duration, frequency, and context of the dissociative disorder contain crucial first-hand data.
- *Psychosocial Assessment.* The fundamental source of the anxiety should be identified as early as possible. Strategies include those effective for recovering unconscious content, such as free association or dream description. At times more active strategies are used, including projective psychometric tests (Rorschach, Thematic Apperception) and hypnosis or intravenous sodium thiopental (Pentothal).
- *Family Counseling.* Inclusion of family members in the therapeutic relationship may be indicated to help them learn new ways to deal with the client.

- *Environmental Manipulation.* It may be necessary to assist the client in problem solving with the goal of minimizing other stressful aspects of the environment.
- *Supportive Insight Therapy.* Clients in whom dissociative phenomena arise primarily against a background of intrapsychic or subjective conflict may benefit from longer-term therapy aimed at surfacing and integrating traumatic experiences and learning new modes of coping with future anxiety.

DOMESTIC VIOLENCE

(*See* Family Violence)

DOUBLE BIND

Two conflicting communications from someone who is crucial for a person's survival. One message is usually verbal and the other nonverbal.

DOWN'S SYNDROME

A type of developmental disability with a complex of congenital deformities, including defective brain development and mental deficiency. It is characterized by an oriental appearance to the face, which gave rise to the name *mongolism.*

DRAW-A-PERSON TEST

(*See* Psychologic Tests)

DRIVE

In psychoanalytic theory, an impulse to action arising in the id from the organism's biologic and physiologic needs and experienced in consciousness as a feeling, a fantasy, or a need to act. The libidinal and the aggressive drives are those primarily involved in psychologic conflict. Personality theory uses the term *motivation*.

DRUGS

(*See* Appendix **B**)

DRUG ABUSE

A state of chronic intoxication that is detrimental to an individual and that is produced by repeated consumption of a drug. The condition is characterized by (1) an overpowering need to take the drug, (2) a willingness to obtain the drug by any means including illegal ones, (3) a tendency to increase the dose, and (4) dependence on the effects of the drug.
(*See also* Substance Use Disorders)

DRUG USE

Ingestion of a chemical in any manner for its effect on the body. The list below defines terms commonly used in discussing drug use and Table 5 (see page 96) provides a general drug use guide for quick reference.

TERM	DEFINITION	EXAMPLE
Drug use	Ingesting in any manner a chemical for its effect on the body	Taking aspirin for headache
Drug abuse	A state of chronic intoxication detrimental to the individual and produced by repeated consumption of a	Street use of heroin

TERM	DEFINITION	EXAMPLE
	drug. Characterized by	
	1. Overpowering need or desire to take the drug despite social or medical problems	
	2. Willingness to obtain the drug by any means including illegal ones	
	3. Tendency to increase the dose	
	4. Physical dependence on effects of drug	
Drug dependence	Dependence on a drug such that	Regular and increasing use of sedatives and hypnotics like diazepam (Valium)
	1. The body re-requires it to continue functioning	
	2. The body develops a tolerance for it, so the person must	

TERM	DEFINITION	EXAMPLE
	increase the dose	
	3. The body develops physical withdrawal symptoms if the drug is stopped	
	4. The person feels that it is impossible to get along without the drug	

TABLE 5. GENERAL DRUG USE GUIDE FOR QUICK REFERENCE

NAME	SLANG NAME	ROUTE OF ADMINIS-TRATION	DESIRED EFFECTS OR REASONS FOR TAKING DRUG
Alcohol	Booze	Orally: liquid	Relaxation, euphoria, disinhibition, social custom and conformity

DSM III

Abbreviation for the third edition of the *Diagnostic and Statistical Manual of Mental Disorders*, published by the American Psychiatric Association in 1980. The DSM III represents the current state of knowledge about diagnosing mental disorders. It is composed of all the official numerical codes and terms for all recognized mental disorders, along with a comprehensive description of each and specified diagnostic criteria that must be present to make each diagnosis.

The multiaxial framework for client assessment provided by the DSM III requires that the clinician collect data about client adaptive strengths as well as about symptoms or problems. In the DSM-III multiaxial system, each individual is evaluated on five axes, each dealing with a different class of information about the client:

(Text continues on page 116.)

OBJECTIVE SYMPTOMS	UNTOWARD SYMPTOMS AND LONG-TERM EFFECTS	SYMPTOMS OF OVERDOSE	FIRST AID
Variable: irritability; reduction in neuromuscular control (affecting speech, gait, coordination); varying behavioral symptoms ranging from release of inhibitions,	Nausea, vomiting, diarrhea; habituation and addiction; irreversible brain and liver damage; gastritis, ulceration, hemorrhage; severe withdrawal symptoms;	Irregularity of behavior and reduction in neuromuscular control, increasingly leading to stupor and coma. On rare occasions, may exhibit outburst of irra-	Acute alcohol intoxication: strong coffee, warm shower followed by cold shower, forced activity, induced vomiting. Generally, if vital signs are stable, no special measures are *(Continued)*

TABLE 5. GENERAL DRUG USE GUIDE FOR QUICK REFERENCE (Continued)

NAME	SLANG NAME	ROUTE OF ADMINIS- TRATION	DESIRED EFFECTS OR REASONS FOR TAKING DRUG
(Alcohol, Continued)			

OBJECTIVE SYMPTOMS	UNTOWARD SYMPTOMS AND LONG-TERM EFFECTS	SYMPTOMS OF OVERDOSE	FIRST AID
congeniality, and increased self-confidence to increase in depression with macabre affect; warm, flushed skin; drowsiness	death (with blood levels above 600 mg/100 mL or after long-term abuse with complications); crosses placental barrier, affecting infant Withdrawal symptoms in adult (in order of succession): tremors ("shakes"); weakness, profuse perspiration, headache, anorexia, nausea, abdominal cramps, retching and vomiting, flushed face, intense craving for alcohol or sedative, acute alcoholic hallucinations, seizures,	tional, combative, and destructive behavior, known as pathologic intoxication or acute alcoholic paranoid state	indicated. Alcohol coma: a medical emergency. Danger is death from respiratory depression. Maintain patient airway; transport for emergency medical treatment. Pathologic intoxication: Use restraints and transport for medical emergency treatment. Withdrawal and delirium tremens: Hospitalize for regimen of intravenous fluids and electrolytes, observation of vital signs, and general

(Continued)

TABLE 5. GENERAL DRUG USE GUIDE FOR QUICK REFERENCE (Continued)

NAME	SLANG NAME	ROUTE OF ADMINIS- TRATION	DESIRED EFFECTS OR REASONS FOR TAKING DRUG
(Alcohol, continued)			
Ampheta- mines	Wake-ups, pep pills, uppers	Orally: pill, capsule; sub- cutaneously; intravenously	Euphoria, relief of fatigue, increase in alertness, loss of appetite

OBJECTIVE SYMPTOMS	UNTOWARD SYMPTOMS AND LONG-TERM EFFECTS	SYMPTOMS OF OVERDOSE	FIRST AID
	agitated delirium		care.
	Fetal alcohol syndrome: prenatal onset, growth deficiency and developmental delay, numerous systemic complications secondary to birth defects		
	Withdrawal symptoms in infant, beginning with drowsiness and irritability		
Variable: remarkable alertness, pressure of speech, irritability; dry mouth, restlessness, agitation, hyperactivity, rapid flight of ideas, mood	Restlessness, irritability, habituation; insomnia, weight loss to malnutrition, unexplainable fear, possible hallucinations, paranoid psychosis, nausea	Dizziness; tremor, irritability, confusion, hostility and assaultiveness, auditory and visual hallucinations, panic states, chest pain and palpita-	"Bad trip": Talk person down, reduce stimuli, and reduce fever. If large amount has been ingested and person is alert, induce vomiting. Attempt to control

(Continued)

TABLE 5. GENERAL DRUG USE GUIDE FOR QUICK REFERENCE (Continued)

NAME	SLANG NAME	ROUTE OF ADMINIS-TRATION	DESIRED EFFECTS OR REASONS FOR TAKING DRUG
(Amphetamines, continued)			
Benzedrine	Bennies, cartwheels		
Dexedrine	Dexies, Christmas trees		
Methedrine	Crystal, speed, meth		
Barbiturates	Barbs, goof-balls, candy, peanuts, pink ladies, block-busters, downers	Orally: cap-sules or pills; intravenously	Relaxation or sleep, euphoria, disinhibition, "rush" after intravenous injection, antidote to ill effects of other drugs

OBJECTIVE SYMPTOMS	UNTOWARD SYMPTOMS AND LONG-TERM EFFECTS	SYMPTOMS OF OVERDOSE	FIRST AID
swings, loss of appetite, weight loss, aggressiveness, increased pulse and blood pressure, dilated pupils, needle marks and tracks with intravenous use	and vomiting, twitching muscles, seizures, hyperpyrexia Withdrawal symptoms: psychic depression, lethargy, apathy, somnolence, lack of initiative; pressure to take amphetamines; suicidal ideation	tions, headache, cardiac arrhythmias, flushed skin, hypertension, vomiting; abdominal cramps, excessive sweating, hyperthermia, shock, convulsions; death	hyperthermia as soon as detected to avoid associated convulsions. With severe physical or behavioral symptoms, immediately seek emergency treatment. Withdrawal: Stay with person and watch for indications of suicidal intent. Seek medical attention.
Variable: relaxation, sometimes euphoria, drowsiness, impaired judgment and coordination, muscle relaxa-	Irritability; weight loss, habituation and addiction, severe withdrawal symptoms, cellulitis and vascular complica-	Slurred speech; staggering gait; sustained nystagmus; slowed reactions; lethargy; progressive respiratory	Overdose: keep person awake and moving to reduce chance of coma. May give activated charcoal to delay (Continued)

TABLE 5. GENERAL DRUG USE GUIDE FOR QUICK REFERENCE (Continued)

NAME	SLANG NAME	ROUTE OF ADMINIS-TRATION	DESIRED EFFECTS OR REASONS FOR TAKING DRUG
(Barbiturates, continued)			
Amytal	Rainbows, blue heavens, blue devils		
Nembutal	Yellow jackets, dolls, abbotts, blockbusters, nemmies		
Phenobarbital	Phennies, purple hearts		
Seconal	Reds, red birds, red devils, pinks		
Tuinal	Rainbows, tuies		

OBJECTIVE SYMPTOMS	UNTOWARD SYMPTOMS AND LONG-TERM EFFECTS	SYMPTOMS OF OVERDOSE	FIRST AID
tion. Pupils may be dilated, but if used in combination with opiates may be pinpoint.	tions after intravenous use, medical dangers inherent with any nonmedical use of hypodermic needles, overdose Withdrawal symptoms in adult: anxiety, sleep disturbances, restlessness, irritability, postural hypotension, tremors, muscular weakness, delirium, seizures, hyperpyrexia Withdrawal symptoms in infant: high-pitched cry, tremors, restlessness, sleep disturbances, hyper-reflexia, hyperphagia, diarrhea, vomiting, seizures	depression evidenced by shallow and irregular breathing; coma; death	gastric absorption. Apply general supportive measures, such as maintaining airway and adequate respirations. Keep warm. Do not use stimulants, because they can cause additional hazards. Transport as soon as possible for emergency medical treatment. Withdrawal: almost invariably requires hospitalization. Transfer for emergency treatment, especially with more advanced symptoms.

(Continued)

105

TABLE 5. GENERAL DRUG USE GUIDE FOR QUICK REFERENCE (Continued)

NAME	SLANG NAME	ROUTE OF ADMINIS-TRATION	DESIRED EFFECTS OR REASONS FOR TAKING DRUG
Cocaine	Coke, snow, big C	Intranasally ("sniffing"), subcutane-ously, intra-venously	Euphoria, to get high, sex-ual stimu-lation
Glue, gaso-line, solvents		Inhalation	To get high, euphoria, relief from depression, increase in sensory awareness
Hallucino-gens			"Mind expansion"; selfexplora-tion, increase

TABLE 5. GENERAL DRUG USE GUIDE FOR QUICK REFERENCE (Continued)

NAME	SLANG NAME	ROUTE OF ADMINIS- TRATION	DESIRED EFFECTS OR REASONS FOR TAKING DRUG	OBJECTIVE SYMPTOMS	UNTOWARD SYMPTOMS AND LONG- TERM EFFECTS	SYMPTOMS OF OVERDOSE	FIRST AID
(Hallucinogens, continued)				Variable: same visions and halluci- nations as amphetamine but for shor- ter periods of time	Hallucina- tions, para- noid thoughts, toxic psycho- sis, scars and abscesses if injected, depression and apathy after a high	Same as for ampheta- mines	Overdose or toxic psycho- sis: Trans- port to medi- cal emer- gency setting immediately.
LSD	Sugar, acid, trip, big D	Orally: liq- uid, capsule, pill (or sugar cube)					
Mescaline	Big chief, mese, pink wedge	Orally: cap- sule, chewing plant		Variable: euphoria, impaired coordination and judg- ment, mood change, slurred speech, impulsive destructive behavior. Effects are brief.	Anorexia, tinnitus, sneezing, coughing, nausea and vomiting, diarrhea, chest pain, muscular and joint pain, visual or auditory hal- lucinations, unconscious- ness. Some substances can severely damage liver or kidneys.	Uncon- sciousness, hypoxia. Death may occur if per- son becomes unconscious and con- tinues to sniff fumes from plastic bag around mouth and nose that maintains airtight seal.	Overdose: Give imme- diate artifi- cial respira- tion with subsequent cardiopulmo- nary resusci- tation (CPR) as indicated. Transfer for medical evaluation.
Peyote	Cactus, bad seed, moon, button						
Psilocybin	Mushrooms			Unusual sen- sations and changes in self-percep-	Anxiety; nausea; chills, trem- ors, shiver-	With large doses or combinations of drugs,	"Bad trip": person needs nonthreaten- ing environ-

(Continued)

TABLE 5. GENERAL DRUG USE GUIDE FOR QUICK REFERENCE (Continued)

NAME	SLANG NAME	ROUTE OF ADMINIS-TRATION	DESIRED EFFECTS OR REASONS FOR TAKING DRUG	OBJECTIVE SYMPTOMS	UNTOWARD SYMPTOMS AND LONG-TERM EFFECTS	SYMPTOMS OF OVERDOSE	FIRST AID
(Hallucinogens, continued)			in visual images and sensory awareness, increase in creativity and insight	tion, occa-sionally hal-lucinations, feelings of euphoria and excitement, rapid mood swings, flight of ideas, sense of observing while parti-cipating, sense of tremen-dous insight. Usual effects are sympa-thomimetic, including pupil dila-tion and increased blood pressure	ing; impaired coordination; rapid mood swings; can precipitate or intensify an existing psy-chosis; depression. "Bad trip" if panic reac-tion occurs with feelings of fear, loss of control, and paranoid mistrust and suspicious-ness. Combi-nations of drugs may lead to depressed level of con-sciousness, seizures, or threatening delusional behavior	seizures or coma may complicate existing anx-iety-provok-ing feelings.	ment with subdued and pleasant stim-uli. Find out from user or friends nature and quantity of drug and time ingested. Maintain understand-ing yet firm approach without cr cal or jud mental a tude. Approa consist talking the pe and s inclu frie oth for pl ta h v

OBJECTIVE SYMPTOMS	UNTOWARD SYMPTOMS AND LONG-TERM EFFECTS	SYMPTOMS OF OVERDOSE	FIRST AID
			Overdose: With overdose or evidence of other complication, including decreased level of consciousness, use supportive measures to maintain airway and immediately transfer to emergency treatment setting. Use of tranquilizing drugs should be avoided if possible. *(Continued)*

TABLE 5. GENERAL DRUG USE GUIDE FOR QUICK REFERENCE (Continued)

NAME	SLANG NAME	ROUTE OF ADMINIS- TRATION	DESIRED EFFECTS OR REASONS FOR TAKING DRUG
Heroin	Smack, "H," horse, junk, shit	Intranasally ("snorting"), orally, intravenously	Euphoria; "thrill," "kick," or "flash"' likened to sexual orgasm with intravenous use

OBJECTIVE SYMPTOMS	UNTOWARD SYMPTOMS AND LONG-TERM EFFECTS	SYMPTOMS OF OVERDOSE	FIRST AID
Foggy period of mental clouding and little inclination toward physical activity; look of sublime contentment with loss of anxiety, worry, sexual desire, appetite; needle tracks; scarred veins; inflammation and edema of nasal mucosa (if snorted)	Itching and decreased blood pressure after intravenous use; habituation and addiction; minimal or absent sexual desire; hepatitis; sepsis; shock; pulmonary edema; allergic reactions; crosses placental barrier, affecting infant Withdrawal symptoms in adult: anxiety; runny nose; dilated pupils; cramps, diarrhea, vomiting, shaking, chills; profuse sweating; sleep disturbances; aches and pains Withdrawal symptoms in	Depressed level of consciousness; depressed respiratory rate; pupillary constriction (unless in combination with other drugs or during anoxic state); pale, cool, clammy skin with cyanotic tinge	Overdose: Immediate support for vital functions is imperative. Institute CPR and transfer to emergency treatment. Withdrawal: Person with beginning symptoms should be seen by physician for medical regimen of methadone or other drugs for symptoms, including control of gastrointestinal symptoms, anxiety, and sleep problems. Person with severe symptoms will need immediate emergency treatment with methadone, pheno- (Continued)

TABLE 5. GENERAL DRUG USE GUIDE FOR QUICK REFERENCE (Continued)

NAME	SLANG NAME	ROUTE OF ADMINIS-TRATION	DESIRED EFFECTS OR REASONS FOR TAKING DRUG
(Heroin, continued)			
Marijuana	Pot, dope, joint, grass, mary jane, boo, charge, hay, jive, sweet lucy, tea, weed, reefer	Inhalation (smoking), orally	Euphoria; to get high, relaxation, social custom or confor-mity, disin-hibition, relief from anxiety or depression, increase in visual and sensory awareness, increase in pleasure dur-ing sexual activity

OBJECTIVE SYMPTOMS	UNTOWARD SYMPTOMS AND LONG-TERM EFFECTS	SYMPTOMS OF OVERDOSE	FIRST AID
	infant: irritability, hyperactivity; tremulousness, vomiting, poor food intake, diarrhea, fever, high-pitched cry; seizures		barbital, and other drugs to alleviate symptoms.
Variable: possible impairment of judgment and coordination, disorientation to time, sense of well-being and tranquility, euphoria, increased appetite (munching), increased pulse, increased awareness of environment	Few symptoms reported: panic reaction with feelings of loss of control or sense of dying, acute depression, toxic psychosis	Same as untoward reaction with feelings of loss of control or depression, may experience nausea and vomiting with oral ingestion	Panic reaction: Use the technique of talking down described under hallucinogen and amphetamine use. Acute depression and psychosis: usually subsides when THC (psychoactive compound in marijuana and hashish) is metabolized. Overdose: Same as above.

Axis I: Clinical syndromes

Conditions not attributable to a mental disorder that are a focus of attention or treatment (V Codes)

Additional codes

Axis II: Personality disorders

Specific developmental disorders

Axis III: Physical disorders

Axis IV: Severity of psychosocial stressors

Axis V: Highest level of adaptive functioning past year

(*See also* Appendix **E**)

DYNAMICS

An explanation of forces (usually unconscious) that are presumed to be at work in a client and that result in the particular symptoms or manifestations observed.

DYSTONIC REACTION

An early, dramatic, extrapyramidal reaction to treatment with antipsychotic medication occurring in the first days of treatment. Characterized by bizarre and severe muscle contractions, usually of the face, tongue, or extraoccular muscles, producing torticollis, opisthotonos, and occulogyric crises. Readily reversible with the use of antiparkinsonian agents.

E

ECHOLALIA
Repetition of another person's words or phrases. Most frequently seen in schizophrenia, particularly the catatonic type.

ECHOPRAXIA
Imitation of another person's movements. Most frequently seen in catatonic schizophrenia.

ECT
(See Electroconvulsive Therapy)

EEG
(See Electroencephalogram)

EGO
A theoretical construct of the organized part of the personality structure that includes defensive, perceptual, intellectual-cognitive, and executive functions. Conscious awareness resides in the ego, although not all operations of the ego are conscious.

EGO-DYSTONIC
Distressing to the individual. For example, neurotic disorders are said to be ego-dystonic.

EGO FUNCTIONS
The functions of self-regulation, balance maintenance, and integrity preservation. They include perception, control of voluntary movement, management of memory, production of adaptive delay between per-

ception and action, choice between "fight" or "flight," selection of needs to be gratified, judging and evaluating internal and external conditions, problem solving, learning, and reality testing.

EGOSYNTONIC

In harmony with one's sense of self. For example, personality disorders are said to be egosyntonic.

ELDERLY

(*See* Aged Persons)

ELECTROCONVULSIVE THERAPY (ECT)

A treatment, generally for depression, that uses electric current to induce unconsciousness and convulsive seizures. There is much controversy concerning its use.

Indications

- Major depression with melancholia (especially in the presence of severe suicidal risk)
- Acute catatonic excitement or severe catatonic withdrawal
- Unipolar or bipolar affective disorders or acute schizophrenia after failure to respond to appropriate trials of psychotropic medication
- In some cases, organic mental syndrome with psychosis secondary to atherosclerosis or senility

Symptoms that predict a good response to ECT:

Feeling of worthlessness

Feeling of helplessness

Feeling of hopelessness

Anorexia

Recent weight loss

Constipation

Reduced libido

Early morning awakening

Suicidal inclinations

Nursing Intervention

- Checking chart for relevant laboratory and physical examination data and for signed consent form
- Seeing that client has nothing by mouth after midnight (for morning treatment) and encouraging client to void
- Checking that hairpins and dentures are removed and that client is dressed in pajamas or other loose clothing
- Having emergency equipment and oxygen available
- Taking client's vital signs
- Observing client after treatment for signs of respiratory difficulties until he or she is fully oriented, alert, and able to get out of bed.

Treatment

For depression, a relatively short course of ECT often brings dramatic results. Clients may respond after 3 or 4 treatments but usually receive 2 or 3 more for a more complete effect. Clients with acute schizophrenia may also respond to a few treatments but require from 10 to 20 to prevent immediate relapse. In all cases, there are no guarantees against eventual relapse.

Complications include memory impairment. (Most investigators believe this to be short term.) Unilateral ECT decreases memory impairment and confusion, but it is not as effective as bilateral ECT. Brain tumor is an absolute contraindication because of increased intracranial pressure. ECT may be used, with caution, in clients who have cardiovascular disease, peptic ulcers, or glaucoma.

ELECTROENCEPHALOGRAM (EEG)
A method of tracing and recording the electrical activity of the brain.

ELECTROSLEEP THERAPY
A treatment mode for schizophrenic, anxious, or depressed persons in which low milliamperage, pulsed, unidirectional current is passed through electrodes placed over the orbits and mastoid processes. Sleep does not actually occur. Treatments are aimed at relieving anxiety, insomnia, and depression. Treatments last ½–1 hour and are given daily in a series of 5 to 10 sessions. The process causes some tingling sensations but no untoward effects.

ELOPEMENT
The departure or flight of a client from a psychiatric hospital without the consent of the staff.

EMOTION
(See Affect)

EMPATHY
The ability to feel the feelings of other people so that one can respond to and understand their experiences on their terms. It is differentiated from sympathy in that empathy does not contain elements of condolence, agreement, or pity.

STEPS IN THERAPEUTIC EMPATHIZING

1. *Identification:* Through relaxation of conscious controls, we allow ourselves to become absorbed in

contemplating the client and the client's experiences.

2. *Incorporation:* We take in the experiences of the client rather than attributing our own experiences and feelings to the client.

3. *Reverberation:* We interplay the internalized feelings of the client and our own experiences or fantasies. While fully absorbed in the identity of the client, we still experience ourselves as separate personalities.

4. *Detachment:* We withdraw from subjective involvement and totally resume our own identities. We use the insight gained from the reverberation phase as well as reason and objectivity to offer responses that are useful to the client.

ENCOPRESIS

Soiling. In the older child, it is rarely physiologic but is the child's expression of anger or hostility. It is usually directed toward the parent with whom the child is experiencing conflict. Interventions include medical evaluation, then assessment and intervention in the parent-child relationship. Therapy may be indicated for child and possibly for parent.

ENCOUNTER GROUP

A form of sensitivity training that emphasizes experiencing individual relationships within the group and that minimizes intellectual and didactic input. The focus is on the present rather than the past or outside problems of group members.

ENDOCRINE DISORDERS

A large number of disorders of endocrine functioning are intertwined with psychological factors. Studying the endocrine system has particular significance for psychiatry because there is a close relationship between the emotions and a variety of neurohumoral processes. In physical medicine, the feedback loop has long been accepted as the model for the functioning of the endocrine organs. (See Table 6, page 124.)

NORMAL DEVELOPMENTAL ALTERATIONS IN ENDOCRINE FUNCTION

DEVELOPMENT	PHYSICAL EVIDENCE	PSYCHOLOGIC ASPECTS
Puberty	Age, growth spurt, changes in fat and muscle proportions and distribution, changes in genitals, changes in secondary sex characteristics, menarche	Changes in popularity, prestige, self-confidence; increase in moodiness, hostility, depression, interpersonal difficulties
Menstruation	Menstrual bleeding cycles, cramps, backaches, headaches, alterations in estrogen: progesterone ratio	Irritability, mood swings, tension, depression
Postpartum	Pregnancy and delivery, vast prior increases in progesterone and estrogen levels during pregnancy fall to normal within ten days, changes in fluid	Emotional lability, body image changes, self-esteem issues, anxiety about adequacy as mother, sensitivity to father's responses to

DEVELOPMENT	PHYSICAL EVIDENCE	PSYCHOLOGIC ASPECTS
	and electrolyte balance, increased prolactin secretion	mother and baby
Menopause	Cessation or irregularity of menses, hot flashes, low levels of estrogen secretion	Anxiety, depression, irritability, decreased sexual interest, end of reproductive era, increased physical illness, loss of youth, issues of children being grown, parents dead or infirm, husband changing

ENURESIS

Ordinarily refers to urinating while asleep (nocturnal enuresis) though some enuretic children wet themselves during the day also. Enuresis is a symptom, not a diagnosis or disease entity. The child under 4 years old is usually not considered enuretic. Causative factors are thought to be faulty toilet training (especially if the child wets during the day also) or psychological stress. Physiologic etiology, such as genitourinary tract infections or central nervous system disease, is rare.

Many approaches to enuresis have been tried, with varying degrees of success. These include imipramine (Tofranil), fluid restriction, behavioral intervention (in which a buzzer wakes the child who is starting to

TABLE 6. DISEASE-INDUCED ALTERATIONS IN ENDOCRINE FUNCTIONS

DISEASE	PHYSICAL SYMPTOMS	MENTAL SYMPTOMS	DIAGNOSTIC TEST
Cushing's syndrome (adrenal cortex hyperfunction)	Truncal obesity, moon faces, abdominal striae, hirsutism, amenorrhea, hypertension, osteoporosis, weakness	Impotence, decreased libido, anxiety, increased emotional lability, apathy, insomnia, memory deficits, confusion, disorientation	Increased 17-hydroxy-corticosteroids
Addison's disease (adrenal insufficiency)	Weakness, fatigue, anorexia, weight loss, nausea and vomiting, pigmentation of skin, hypotension	Depression, irritability, psychomotor retardation, apathy, memory defect, hallucinations	Decreased urinary steroids; decreased sodium chlorides, bicarbonates; increased potassium
Hyperthyroidism	Staring, exophthamos, goiter, moist warm skin, weight loss, increased appetite, weakness, tremor, tachycardia, heat intolerance	Anxiety, tension, irritability, hyperexcitability, emotional lability, depression, psychosis, or delirium	Increased protein-bound iodine (PBI); increased T_3, T_4; increased radioactive iodine uptake
Hypothyroidism	Dull expression, puffy	Psychomotor retarda-	Decreased PBI, decreased

	eyelids, swollen tongue, hoarse voice, rough dry skin, cold intolerance	tion, decreased initiative, slow comprehension, drowsiness, decreased recent memory, delirium, stupor, depression or psychosis	thyroid symptoms, increased cholesterol, hypochromic anemia
Diabetes mellitus	Polydipsia, polyuria, polyphagia, weight loss, blurred vision, fatigue, impotence, fainting, paresthesia	Stupor, coma, fatigue, impotence	Increased fasting blood sugar, increased 2-hour postprandial, abnormal glucose tolerance test
Hypoglycemia	Tremor, light-headedness, sweating, hunger, nausea, pallor, tachycardia, hypertension	Anxiety, fugure, unusual behavior, confusion, apathy, psychomotor agitation or retardation, depression, delusions, hallucinations, convulsions, coma	Abnormal glucose tolerance test

wet), and psychotherapy. Educating parents in bladder-training techniques and attitudes can help solve the problem on a primary level. It is important when working with enuretic children or their parents to help the child overcome feelings of shame and guilt. These feelings are often exacerbated by well-meaning but misguided parents.

EPILEPSY

A disorder characterized by periodic, recurring, short-lived disturbances of consciousness such as seizures or convulsions. It may have no apparent organic basis, or it may be due to organic lesions. (See Table 7.)

(See also Organic Brain Syndrome)

EXCESSIVE DEPENDENCE

(See Learned Helplessness)

TABLE 7. TYPES OF EPILEPSY

TYPE	AGE OF ONSET	SIGNS AND SYMPTOMS	ELECTROENCEPHALOGRAM ABNORMALITY BETWEEN SEIZURES
Generalized Grand mal	1–15 years	Aura, unconsciousness, tonic-clonic seizure	20% abnormal awake 40% abnormal asleep
Petit mal	5 years	No aura, 2–15-second lapse of consciousness, blinking, twitching	85% abnormal awake 90% abnormal asleep
Focal Jacksonian	Often post-traumatic	Begins in thumb or face, motor or sensory march of symptoms	30% abnormal awake 60% abnormal asleep
Psychomotor	20 years	Behavior and personality changes, lip-smacking	20% abnormal awake 80% abnormal asleep
Other	1–6 years	Aura, focal movements or twitching related to localization	20% abnormal awake 80% abnormal asleep
Hypothalamic	15 years	Rage attacks; emotional, sensory, and vegetative aura	8% abnormal awake 90% abnormal asleep

F

FACILITATIVE COMMUNICATION
Communication that aims at initiating, building, and maintaining fulfilling and trusting relationships with other persons.

(See Appendix **C**, Skills that Foster Effective Communication)

FACTITIOUS DISORDERS
Factitious means not genuine or natural. In DSM III, this category of disorders includes conditions in which a client has physical or psychological symptoms that are actually produced by the client under conscious, voluntary control. Clients who have factitious disorders may produce a symptom like hematuria (blood in their urine) by taking anticoagulants or self-induce a dislocation of the shoulder for no other reason than to assume a patient role. The distinction between factitious and somatoform disorders is that the physical symptoms present are under voluntary control in factitious disorders and not under voluntary control in somatoform disorders. Both conditions must be thoughtfully assessed for the possible presence of a true physical disorder.

FAILURE TO THRIVE
(See Reactive Attachment Disorder of Infancy)

FAMILY THERAPY
Psychotherapy in which all, or almost all, members of a family system participate at once. Family therapy is

a different way of viewing problems. In general, family therapists believe that the emotional symptoms or problems of an individual are an expression of emotional symptoms or problems of a family. Therefore, the family system is viewed as the basic unit of treatment. The concerns of family therapists are basically with the relationships between the family members, not with the intrapsychic functioning of individuals.

Assessment

■ Identification of the family life issue, its effects on family functioning, and the affect that accompanies it. Is the issue the basics of life, such as food, shelter, or money; the entry of a third person; the exit of children from the household; illness?

■ Identification of the assets, liabilities, and capabilities of the family in terms of resolving the issue and coping with the accompanying affects. What are the nature and effectiveness of each member's defense mechanisms, cognitive capacities, and communicative abilities?

■ Identification of the willingness and ability of family members to undertake therapeutic tasks. Is the family willing to participate? Is it able to change?

Treatment

Family therapists often reverse the traditional territorial control of the professional by engaging the family system in therapy in its own milieu—the home. There are several reasons for this: (1) the interactions of the family system are more natural in their usual environment; (2) customary roles are played out more spontaneously on home ground; (3) family members reluctant to participate in therapy tend to be less so in the home than in a formal office or mental health agency setting.

Goal negotiation is an important phase in family therapy. Each member is asked to identify what she or he would like to see changed in the family. When each member and the therapist have identified what they see as important goals, compromise is needed to achieve a working goal for the entire family.

FAMILY TIME LINE
A family genealogy or tracing that serves as a limited means for understanding a family's roots.

FAMILY VIOLENCE
Gained attention in the 1970s as a social problem of magnitude. Before that time the beating of children, wives, and the elderly was often justified as necessary discipline.

Battered Women

Stereotypes continue to exist. Three common stereotypes are:

Battered women are basically sadomasochistic.

Battered women actually instigate assaults: If they would stop nagging and insulting their husbands, their husbands would stop beating them.

Battered women are "castrating females," domineering women who exploit their husbands.

These stereotypes place blame on the victim and support the beating of women by men as part of the masculine mystique.

Considerations

- Battered women tend not to leave their battering spouses as they feel ill-prepared to meet the financial needs that would face them if they lived alone or are concerned that their husbands will cause them even greater harm.

- Battered women tend not to report the crime to the police because they are intimidated by threats of further physical violence. (Also, the police officer's suggestion to "kiss and makeup" seldom works.)
- Domestic violence may escalate to murder by either party.

Child Abuse

Preconditions for child abuse include:

1. The presence of potential within the family, which includes:
   a. Parents reared in a physically or emotionally traumatic manner
   b. Parents who are isolated and distrustful
   c. Parents who give each other little help
   d. Parents who have a poor self-image
   e. Parents who have unrealistic expectations of children
2. The presence of a special child who
   a. Is seen as different
   b. Really is different
   c. Is both different and seen as different
3. The presence of a crisis or crises that are
   a. Physical (no food, money, heat, lights)
   b. Personal (death, separation)
   c. Both physical and personal

- While one child may be identified as different and is therefore the target of parental abuse, the nurse assessing the family should carefully consider siblings as potential, if not yet actual, victims.
- Child abuse, like poverty and racism, is a vicious circle: Abused children frequently become abusive parents. Knowing this enables the nurse to maintain

an empathic attitude when dealing with battering parents.
- The health professional who blames the battering parents will only compound the problem by intensifying these feelings and making the parent more resistant to intervention.

Intervention

1. Most abusive parents can be helped; this involves learning a new pattern of parenting.
2. Intervention strategies include personal therapy for the parent, support groups, group therapy, parenting classes, and the development of a support system.
3. Family Therapy is viewed by many mental health professionals as the most effective single intervention in working with battering families. Family therapists:
   a. Must be in touch with their own feelings about child abuse and abusive parents
   b. Must recognize that battering parents have many of the same needs as their children—primarily severe and unmet dependency needs
   c. Must be able to accept the parents as worthwhile persons

Nursing Intervention

- Refer to local protective services all cases of confirmed or suspected child abuse.
- Be alert for potentially abusive parents (such as those who experienced childhood deprivation and are now under stress) and attempt primary prevention.
- Talk about the problem of battering parents and child abuse; use opportunities in professional and private life to share information about it.

- Be aware of own feelings about child abuse and battering parents.
- Be honest and empathic when dealing with abusive parents.

FANTASY

A defense mechanism that is a sequence of mental images, like a daydream. It may be conscious or unconscious. It is considered by some to be an individual's attempt to resolve an emotional conflict. Fantasy is a form of nonrational mental activity that enables the individual to escape temporarily the demands of the everyday world. Fantasies are not confined by the reality considerations of cause and effect and time and space.

Fantasy normally characterizes the thinking of children before they are able to engage in consensually validated communication. Adults revert to fantasy during times of stress to obtain a symbolic satisfaction of wishes. Fantasy may offer temporary relief from pressure, but people who spend too much time in fantasy may be unable to meet the requirements of reality.

(*See also* Defense Mechanisms)

FEEDBACK

The process by which performance is checked and malfunctions corrected; a regulatory function in the communication process, requiring two persons—one to give it and one to receive it.

(*See also* Appendix **C**, Skills That Foster Effective Communication)

FLASHBACKS

Hallucinogenic drug induced visual distortions (intense colors, trails, geometric forms in objects) or an experience of reliving intense emotions that occurred during a previous drug experience. Both kinds of flash-back are more likely to occur when the person is under-going stress or is falling asleep. These are times when ego functions are somewhat disturbed, making the person susceptible to invasion by feelings.

(*See also* Drug Use; Substance Use Disorder)

FLIGHT OF IDEAS
A state in which thoughts come so quickly and bring so many associations that no single thought can be clearly expressed. The person's ideas occur in a rapid and endless variety with only a single, slim thread connecting them.

(*See also* Mental Status Examination)

FOLIE À DEUX
A condition in which two closely related people exhibit nearly identical psychopathologic conditions.

FORENSIC PSYCHIATRY
The branch of psychiatry that deals with the legal aspects of psychiatric disorders.

FREE ASSOCIATION
A psychoanalytic technique whereby a patient says whatever comes to mind.

FUGUE (PSYCHOGENIC)
Persons with this disorder wander—usually far from home and for days at a time—completely forgetting their past lives and associations. Unlike people with amnesia, they are unaware of having forgotten any-thing. When they return to their former consciousness, they are amnesic for the period covered by the fugue. Fugue clients are generally seclusive and quiet, and as

a consequence, their behavior rarely attracts attention.

(See also Dissociative Disorders)

FUNCTIONAL
Having a psychologic rather than an organic (physical) cause.

G

GENERAL ADAPTATION SYNDROME

The objectively measurable structural and chemical changes produced in the body when stress affects the whole body, this syndrome occurs in three stages:

1. Alarm
2. Resistance
3. Exhaustion

GENERALIZED ANXIETY DISORDER

In this syndrome anxiety is not displaced or automatically controlled by some repetitive thought or act. Instead, it remains diffuse, free floating and painful.

Symptoms of Generalized Anxiety Disorder

PHYSIOLOGIC	EMOTIONAL	INTELLECTUAL
Increased heart rate	Irritability	Forgetfulness
Elevated blood pressure	Angry outbursts	Preoccupation
Tightness of chest	Feeling of worthlessness	Rumination
Difficulty in breathing	Depression	Mathematical and grammatical errors
Sweaty palms	Suspiciousness	Errors in judging distance
Trembling, tics, or twitching	Jealousy	Blocking
Tightness of neck or back	Restlessness	Diminished fantasy life
	Anxiousness	Lack of concentration
	Withdrawal	
	Diminished initiative	

PHYSIOLOGIC	EMOTIONAL	INTELLECTUAL
muscles	Tendency to cry	Lack of attention to detail
Headache	Sobbing without tears	Past rather than present- or future-orientation
Urinary frequency		
Diarrhea	Reduced personal involvement with others	
Nausea and/or vomiting		Lack of awareness of external stimuli
Sleep disturbance	Tendency to blame others	Reduced creativity
Anorexia	Excessive criticism of self and others	Diminished productivity
Sneezing		
Constant state of fatigue		Reduced interest
Accident proneness	Self-deprecation	
Susceptibility to minor illness	Lack of interest	
Slumped posture		

(*See also* Anxiety)

GERIATRIC

(*See* Aged Persons)

GESTALT THERAPY

A type of psychotherapy that emphasizes treatment of the person as a whole—biologic component parts and their organic functioning, perceptual configuration, and interrelationships with the outside world. Focuses on sensory awareness of here-and-now experiences rather than on past recollections or future expectations.

GRANDEUR, DELUSIONS OF

(See Delusions)

GRIEF WORK/GRIEVING

A response to a loss, usually of a loved person through death or separation, but grieving also follows the loss of anything, tangible or intangible, that is highly valued: a material possession, a position of status, a body part, a home, or a country. An understanding of the reactions common to loss in general will help in understanding grief reactions to the death of a loved person.

Normal Grief Reactions

Although painful, grieving is important. The following list identifies five general classes of symptoms of normal grief.

SYMPTOM CLASSIFICATION	CHARACTERISTICS
1. Somatic distress	Occurs in waves lasting from 20 minutes to 1 hour
	Deep, sighing respirations most common when discussing grief
	Lack of strength
	Loss of appetite and sense of taste
	Tightness in throat
	Choking sensation

SYMPTOM CLASSIFICATION	CHARACTERISTICS
	accompanied by shortness of breath
2. Preoccupation with image of deceased	Similar to daydreaming
	May mistake others for deceased person
	May be oblivious to surroundings
	Slight sense of unreality
	Fear of becoming "insane"
3. Feelings of guilt	Accuses self of negligence
	Exaggerates existence and importance of negative thoughts, feelings, and actions toward deceased
	Views self as having failed deceased—"If I had only. . . ."
4. Feelings of hostility	Irritability, anger, and loss of warmth toward others
	May attempt to handle feelings of hostility in formalized and stiff manner of social interaction
5. Loss of patterns of conduct	Inability to initiate or maintain organized patterns of activity

**SYMPTOM
CLASSIFICATION**

CHARACTERISTICS

Restlessness, with aimless movements

Loss of zest—tasks and activities are carried on as though with great effort

Activities formerly carried on in company of deceased have lost their significance

May become strongly dependent on whoever stimulates mourner to activity

Morbid Grief Reactions

When a person attempts to handle normal but uncomfortable grief symptoms by avoiding encounters with others and increasing interpersonal distance or deliberately excluding from the thinking process all references to the deceased, a morbid grief reaction may result.

Morbid grief reactions include:

**SYMPTOM
CLASSIFICATION**

CHARACTERISTICS

1. Delayed reaction

Most common and most dramatic morbid reaction

Postponement may be brief or prolonged for years

SYMPTOM CLASSIFICATION	CHARACTERISTICS
	Usually occurs when bereaved is confronted with necessity of carrying out important tasks or maintaining morale of others
2. Distorted reactions	Excessive activity with no sense of loss
	Development of physical symptoms similar to those experienced by deceased just before death
	Medical illness of psychophysiologic nature, developed close in time to loss of important person
	Continued and progressive social isolation with alteration in relationships with friends and relatives
	Extreme hostility against specific persons somehow connected with death event
	"Schizophreniclike" wooden and formal

SYMPTOM CLASSIFICATION	CHARACTERISTICS
	conduct, masking hostile feelings
	Lasting change in patterns of social interaction
	Activities detrimental to own social and economic existence
	Agitated depression

Successful grieving usually consists of the following three stages:

1. *Shock and Disbelief.* Characterized as the "Oh, No!" stage; the need to deny loss is paramount. Behavior may run gamut from verbal denial to incapacitation and reflects attempts by bereaved persons to protect themselves from recognition and/or pain evoked by the event. Denial during this phase serves a therapeutic purpose. It protects bereaved people from painful knowledge with which they may be unable to cope. Continued denial, however, signals distress. A therapeutic maneuver that may be helpful is an expression of the nurse's own perceptions of the facts of the situation, while avoiding arguments based on logic.

2. *Developing Awareness.* As awareness of loss becomes acute, crying is evident. Tears should not be discouraged, but rather allowed. Anger may be felt toward deceased person for leaving; this may take the form of self-injury or self-destructive behavior. Before giving sedation to grieving persons, consider whether it will facilitate or subvert the grieving process. Do not move in too quickly to

suppress the expression of emotion. The nurse needs to be a good listener who is willing to spend time hearing expression of grief and reminiscences.

3. *Restitution.* This completes the work of mourning and is often assisted by traditional mourning practices; rituals allow supportive interpersonal interactions to occur. Early in the restitution period, the memory of the dead person is elevated to a degree of perfection; it may take many months for the mourner to see the deceased as he or she actually was.

Mourning is frequently completed within the year following the death. However, when the mourner has not experienced all three stages, grieving cannot be considered complete, and some of the work of mourning must still be done.

GROUP PSYCHOTHERAPY

Psychotherapy of several clients at the same time in the same session. It may emphasize examination of the interpersonal relationships of members of the group to see how they usually interact with others. Many types of groups are found in mental health settings or in communities at large. Although specific methods and techniques vary according to the purpose of the group or the skills and theoretic orientation of the therapist, certain common principles seem to apply to all groups. For example, in all therapeutic groups, interaction plays a crucial role in characterologic change.

Questions concerning a prospective group member include:

- What is the person's motivation for therapy?
- What effect will the prospective member have on the others, in terms of his or her ability to bring curative factors into play?

- Does the person's age, occupation, or sex match the others so that the member will not be singled out as different or deviant?
- Is the prospective member similar to the others in terms of his or her vulnerability or ego strength?
- Is the person likely to terminate prematurely?

The group contract identifies the shared rights and responsibilities of therapists and members. It is an agreed set of rules or arrangements for the structure and functioning of the group. It may be written or verbal, and it should cover the following elements:

Goals and purposes of the group

Time and length of meetings

Place of meetings

Starting and ending dates

Addition of new members

Attendance

Confidentiality

Roles of members and therapists

Fees

Tasks of the Therapist

- Steer the group into the here-and-now. Events in the session take precedence over those that occurred outside. As the group progresses, much of the work is taken on by the members.
- Illuminate process; the group must move beyond a focus on content toward a focus on process—that is, the "how" and "why" of an interaction. Process commentary is anxiety producing and may make the therapist vulnerable to criticism and retaliation by others.

Characteristic member behaviors and nursing interventions in phases of group therapy include:

MEMBER BEHAVIOR	NURSING INTERVENTIONS
1. Beginning Phase Anxiety is high	Move to reduce anxiety; avoid making demands until group anxiety has abated
Members unsure of what to do or say; need to be included	Be active and provide some structure and direction; suggest members introduce themselves; work to sustain therapeutic rather than social role; include all members and encourage sharing but limit monopolizing
Members unclear about contract	Clarify contract; give information to dispel confusion or misunderstandings
Members test therapists and other members in terms of trustworthiness, value stances, etc., often through seemingly unimportant issues	Capitalize on opportunity to "pass" tests by proving trustworthy and by being open to and accepting values of others
Beginning attempts at self-disclosure and problem	Focus on related themes; begin exploration; begin to focus on

MEMBER BEHAVIOR	NURSING INTERVENTIONS
identification are made	here-and-now experiences in session
Members have sense of "I"-ness, little sense of "we"-ness	Encourage involvement with others through curative factor of *universality*
2. Middle Phase	Encourage cohesion; provide opportunity for expression of warm feelings
Sense of "I"-ness is replaced by sense of "we"-ness	
Self-disclosure increases	Encourage exploration and move to problem solving
Members are more aware of interpersonal interactions in the here-and-now	Encourage members to participate in observing and commenting on here-and-now; make process comments
Additions and losses of members evoke strong reactions	Prepare members for additions and losses where possible; provide opportunity to talk about addition and loss experience
Ability to maintain focus on one topic increases	Encourage exploration of topic area in depth
3. Termination Phase	Provide adequate time in as many sessions as necessary to work through affective responses; be sure members know termi-
Feelings about separation may run gamut (anger, sadness, indif-	

MEMBER BEHAVIOR	**NURSING INTERVENTIONS**
ference, joy, etc.)	nation date in advance; help members leave with positive feelings by identifying positive changes that have occurred in individual members and in group
Members may feel lost and rudderless	Explore support systems available to individual members; bridge gap where possible (to another agency, another therapist, etc.); keep in focus task of resolving loss

H

HALLUCINATION

A sensory impression in the absence of external stimuli that occurs during the waking state. Visual and auditory hallucinations are the most common in psychiatric conditions. Tactile, olfactory, and gustatory hallucinations are most often related to organic disorders. In psychiatric conditions, tactile, olfactory, gustatory, and kinesthetic hallucinations may be mixed with illusions and delusional systems.

(*See also* Mental Status Examination; Psychotic Disorders)

HALLUCINOGENIC DRUGS

Lysergic acid diethylamide (LSD), mescaline, psilocybin, and tetrahydrocannabinal (THC) are not physically addictive, but they can produce psychologic dependence and tolerance. Some of these drugs, such as LSD, are synthetic. Others, such as mescaline and psilocybin, are contained in certain cactuses and mushrooms, which are important in the spiritual rites of certain Indian cultures in the United States and Mexico. The most characteristic effect of these drugs is a kaleidoscopic visual hallucination of vivid colors and forms. Moods and perceptions may also vary dramatically. The major problems usually associated with use of these drugs are bad trips and flashbacks.

(*See also* Drug Use, Substance Use Disorders)

HEADACHE

Tension headache and other kinds of headache resulting from vascular changes, such as migraine, comprise the group of headaches not related to intracranial lesions, diseases, or either systemic or local infections. Structural or disease-related headaches arise from:

Systemic infections

Primary or metastatic tumors

Hematomas

Abscesses

Cranial infections

Cranial nerve inflammations

Eye, ear, nose, sinus, or tooth diseases

HEPATIC ENCEPHALOPATHY

Damage to liver cells for any reason can cause organic brain changes. Physical signs of liver disease include telangiectasia, ascites, esophageal varices, caput medusae, flapping tremor of hands, and jaundice. Mental status changes range from confusion and apathy to disorientation and psychosis, with coma as a preterminal event.

(See also Organic Brain Syndrome)

HISTORY, PSYCHIATRIC

(See Psychiatric History)

HISTRIONIC PERSONALITY DISORDER

(See Personality Disorders)

HOSPITALIZED CHILD

Hospitalized children of any age are under great stress and need psychiatric nursing interventions. It has been demonstrated in both clinical and research settings that hospitalized children need emotional, as well as physical, care.

Nursing Intervention

The nursing care plans next give the main objectives and interventions for the hospitalized child:

Infant (Birth to 1 Year)

PATIENT CARE OBJECTIVES	NURSING INTERVENTIONS
To help infant develop trust	1. Assign one nurse and one relief staff member to care for infant.
	2. Arrange parental rooming-in, if possible.
	3. Provide infant with a maternal substitute if parent does not room-in.
	4. Encourage parent to participate in care as much as possible.
	5. Have parent present during assigned nurse's first interactions with infant to facilitate infant's trust in nurse.
To provide infant with pleasurable sensory and tactile stimulation	1. Provide cuddly toys and visual stimulants, such as mobiles.
	2. Provide auditory stimulation, such as

**PATIENT CARE
OBJECTIVES**

NURSING INTERVENTIONS

music, singing,
talking

3. Provide tactile stim-
ulation by holding,
cuddling, rocking.

To support
parents so they
can continue to
meet infant's needs

1. Work closely with
parents, giving them
recognition and
helping them to stay
involved in infant's
care.

2. Offer parents the
opportunity to
express their needs
and feelings. (A psy-
chiatric nurse clini-
cian or other mental
health worker could
meet this need.)

3. Ward staff members
should offer parents
the opportunity to
talk and should
accept their possible
frustration, anger, or
fears.

Toddler (1–3 years)

To avoid disrupt-
ing parent-child
relationship, which
toddler needs in

1. Have parent room-in
if possible.

2. Involve parent in
child's care as much

151

PATIENT CARE OBJECTIVES

NURSING INTERVENTIONS

order to accomplish separation-individuation process

as possible.

3. Explain the dynamics of separation anxiety and the toddler's vulnerability to parents. If parents do not understand why the child is clingy or appears to ignore them during visits, they may visit less often.

4. Provide parents with support, so they can continue to support child. Specifically, parents need the opportunity to verbalize feelings, concerns, fears, and anger.

To help toddler meet needs for control

1. Whenever possible, offer a choice, for example, a choice of foods. Do not offer a "choice" concerning necessary medical procedures that the child in fact has no choice about.

2. Be honest and consistent.

PATIENT CARE
OBJECTIVES

NURSING INTERVENTIONS

3. Encourage verbal
and symbolic
expression of con-
flicts to help the
child assimilate and
master frightening
events and feelings.

To help parents
and child separate
when necessary

1. Have parents tell
child when they will
return.

2. Have parents leave
immediately after
they tell child
they're going.

3. Stay with child for
awhile after parents
leave. Let parents
know you will do
this to help child to
cope with their
leaving.

4. Give parents recognition and support
for being able to
separate from child.

5. Stress that it is
important for par-
ents to return when
they tell child they
will. Also stress the
importance of not
lying to the child
("Mommy's just

**PATIENT CARE
OBJECTIVES**

NURSING INTERVENTIONS

going to the store.
I'll be right back") or
leaving without let-
ting child know.

6. Make sure child
knows when parent
will return. Toddlers
do not understand
time well, so relate
visits to daily activ-
ity. For instance,
rather than saying,
"Your mommy will
be back tomorrow at
nine," say, "After
you go to bed, wake
up in the morning,
and eat breakfast,
mommy will be
back."

To help child deal
with fear of aban-
donment

1. Try to incorporate
some of child's home
routines into the
hospital care to give
the child a sense of
stability about some
aspects of daily life.

2. Have parents leave
transitional objects
from home with
child.

3. Promote continuity
of the parent-child

**PATIENT CARE
OBJECTIVES**

NURSING INTERVENTIONS

relationship (see
first objective),
stressing to parents
the importance of
regular visiting if
parents are not
rooming-in.

4. Give child opportun-
ity to use play to
help resolve fears
and conflicts. If
child is nonambula-
tory and cannot go
to the ward play-
room, furnish child
with toys and
companionship.

To prepare child
for medical or
surgical procedures

1. Give toddler oppor-
tunity to play with
as much as possible
of the equipment
used in his or her
care, such as sy-
ringes without
needles.

2. Tell younger toddler
about a procedure
just before it is to be
done. Tell older
toddlers several
hours ahead, or ear-
lier if considerable
preparation is

PATIENT CARE OBJECTIVES

NURSING INTERVENTIONS

involved.

3. Be honest about whether the procedure will hurt.

4. Be clear with child that necessary medical procedures will be carried out and that child doesn't have a choice about them.

5. Encourage child to express objections to and anger about being subjected to painful or frightening procedures and having no control over them. Expression may be verbal or symbolic (through play). Indicate verbally acceptance of child's feelings by saying, for instance, "I guess you're pretty mad at me because I gave you that shot. It's hard to have to get shots."

PATIENT CARE OBJECTIVES

Child (3–6 years)

To help child meet the developmental task of achieving a sense of initiative versus guilt

NURSING INTERVENTIONS

1. Provide the child with some stability by assigning one nurse and one relief staff member to the child.

2. Explain to parents the importance of regular visits. These give children confidence in continued parental support and love that they need to continue to explore themselves and environment.

3. Be aware that the Oedipal-age child is absorbed with guilt and blame and egocentric thinking. When appropriate, stress to these children that no one (including themselves) is to blame for their illness. One strategy to convey this, if the child does not verbalize or

PATIENT CARE
OBJECTIVES

NURSING INTERVENTIONS

otherwise directly
communicate con-
cern, is to say,
"Sometimes kids
think they get sick
because they're bad
or someone is pun-
ishing them. That's
not true."

4. Give the child
opportunity to use
play and play mate-
rials to help resolve
feelings of guilt.
Many children will
play out fantasies
they won't verbalize.
For instance, the
child might have a
doll or toy animal be
sick because "he's
bad." Playtimes are
opportunities for the
nurse to assess the
child's possible feel-
ings of guilt or
blame or both and
offer reassurance.

5. Encourage these
children to partici-
pate in their own
medical and per-
sonal care. This
gives them a sense

**PATIENT CARE
OBJECTIVES**

NURSING INTERVENTIONS

of control, confidence, and mastery.

6. Praise the child for exploring and participating in self-care. Encourage questions and give positive reinforcement for curiosity and for child's ability to understand answers.

To help child deal with mutilation and castration fantasies

1. Before explaining child's condition, find out how child understands it. If child will not verbalize his or her ideas, nurse may be able to assess them during a play session.

2. Be aware that Oedipal-age children tend to believe their entire body is vulnerable. This is especially important in pre-and postoperative teaching. Stress that surgical procedure will be (or was) limited to one specific part of the body.

PATIENT CARE OBJECTIVES

NURSING INTERVENTIONS

3. Give child materials and opportunity to play out, and thus help resolve, mutilation fears.

4. Offer clear explanations of child's condition and treatment.

To prepare child for medical or surgical procedures

1. This age group can understand simple anatomy and physiology, so offer specific explanations, rather than general ones such as, "We are going to fix your eyes."

2. Find out how much child understands about condition and treatments both before and after explaining them. Then clarify misunderstandings and deal with possible fantasies of guilt and mutilation.

3. Use visual aids. These should include body outline drawings, dolls, and actual equipment

PATIENT CARE
OBJECTIVES

NURSING INTERVENTIONS

used in treatment,
such as intravenous
tubing, dressings,
and drains. Encour-
age child to handle
and play with
equipment.

Child (6–12 years)

To help child use
hospitalization to
achieve a sense of
industry by promot-
ing exploration and
mastery of skills

1. Find out how much
   child understands
   about condition.
   Then actively
   involve child as you
   teach about it.

2. When teaching, use
   a more sophisti-
   cated, scientific
   approach than is
   used with younger
   children. Include
   medical terminology.
   Give verbal recogni-
   tion of understand-
   ing and learning.

3. Encourage questions
   and curiosity.

4. Make actual equip-
   ment available to
   child for explora-
   tion. Give verbal
   recognition if child
   is able to use
   equipment.

PATIENT CARE OBJECTIVES	NURSING INTERVENTIONS
To encourage interactions with peers	1. Peer relationships are important in this age group, so encourage peer interaction by strategies such as

    a. Making available a playroom that includes games, interesting equipment or models, and other toys that promote group play.

    b. Involving the nonambulant child by wheeling bed into playroom so that other children can come in to play.

    c. Offering child in isolation more direct contact with nurse.

    d. Teaching about common experiences, such as injections, in a group setting. Use actual equipment and encourage participation.

NURSING INTERVENTIONS

To help child deal
with possible fears
of death

1. Be aware that a fear
of death is common
at this age.

2. Encourage verbal
expression of fears
and symbolic
expression through
play. Child may not
express fear directly
but may tell stories
about children who
died.

3. Be very clear when
teaching about
which part of the
child's body will be
involved. Stress that
no other body part
will be involved.

4. Let child know that
many other children
have been treated
successfully at the
hospital for the
same condition.

5. Express confidence
in child's physician
and in other health
workers.

To prepare child
for medical and
surgical procedures

1. See first part of this
section and section
on preparation of
Oedipal-age child

PATIENT CARE
OBJECTIVES

NURSING INTERVENTIONS

for specific
techniques.

2. Be alert for the pos-
   sibility of regression
   due to the stress of
   hospitalization. This
   stress may arouse
   fears, such as fear of
   separation or mutila-
   tion, normally
   associated with a
   younger age group.

3. Hospitalization is
   usually less trau-
   matic for latency-
   age child, since
   these children
   separate more easily
   from parents and
   home, are interested
   in trying out new
   roles and exploring
   new situations, and
   are more reality
   oriented and better
   able to reason than
   younger child. If
   nurse uses these
   characteristics in
   helping child to cope
   with the hospitaliza-
   tion, it can be a pos-
   itive experience for
   child.

HOSTILITY

Actual or threatened aggressive contact. It is generally differentiated from anger in that hostility is considered to be destructive in intent while anger may be a constructive expression.

The operational steps in direct expression of hostility are:

1. Client experiences a frustration or threat.
2. Anxiety surfaces, associated with feelings of helplessness and inadequacy.
3. Verbal or motor aggressive action alleviates the increased anxiety.

Aggressive action is directed toward destruction of the object perceived as the source of the frustration or threat. This object may be self, others, or an inanimate object. When forces inhibit the direct expression of hostility, the client may cope with the hostility by using various defense mechanisms. Examples include displacement and projection.

(*See also* Aggression: Verbal Threats)

HUNTINGTON'S CHOREA

A hereditary disease with an onset in adult life (ages 25–50), Huntington's chorea is a syndrome of progressive mental deterioration and a jerking movement of the face and limbs.

Assessment

In its incipient stages, the organic mental changes are reflected either in mood disturbances or in impulsive, erratic, or irresponsible behavior. Only in the later stages does dementia develop. In addition to choreiform movements, client has speech difficulties and an ataxic, drunken gait. The family history may confirm the diagnosis, since Huntington's is passed to half the children of an affected parent (it has a dominant role of inheritance).

(*See also* Organic Brain Syndrome)

HYPERACTIVE CHILD

A child in a state of increased rate of activity, which may include emotional lability and flight of ideas.

Assessment

Many children are incorrectly labeled hyperactive. The American Psychiatric Association, in the DSM III, has delineated the following criteria for this diagnosis:

1. Inattention (child demonstrates at least three)
   a. Fails to finish things started
   b. Often doesn't seem to listen
   c. Is easily distracted
   d. Has difficulty concentrating
   e. Has difficulty sticking to play activities
2. Impulsivity (at least three)
   a. Often acts before thinking
   b. Shifts excessively from one activity to another
   c. Has difficulty organizing work
   d. Needs a lot of supervision
   e. Often calls out in class
   f. Has difficulty awaiting turn in games or group situations
3. Hyperactivity (at least two)
   a. Excessively runs about or climbs on things
   b. Has difficulty sitting still
   c. Has difficulty staying seated
   d. Moves about excessively during sleep
   e. Is always "on the go"

(*American Psychiatric Association* 1980, pp. 26-28).

In addition, onset must be before 7 years, symptoms must have lasted at least 6 months, and condition must not be due to another mental disorder. The child suffering from an attention deficit disorder without hyperactivity would display the same symptoms, excepting signs of hyperactivity.

Treatment

Treatment for the child with an attention deficit disorder with hyperactivity is controversial. Sometimes methylphenidate hydrochloride (Ritalin) is prescribed, which for some clinicians raises the issue of whether an individual should be medicated in order to fit more smoothly into the environment. Therapy can help the child decrease anxiety and increase self-esteem, thus reducing the symptoms.

HYPERTENSIVE CRISIS

A side effect of monoamine-oxidase inhibitor drugs which may lead to intracranial bleeding and subsequent death.

(*See also* Appendix **B**, Antidepressant Drugs)

HYPERTHYROIDISM

Psychiatric symptoms can be the most notable abnormalities in a thyrotoxic patient. These may include restlessness, tremulousness, agitation, and acute delirious states. Because it is a hypermetabolic state, hyperthyroidism causes physical changes in many organ systems, making diagnosis easier. Warm moist skin, accelerated heart rate, increased appetite, weight loss, heat intolerance, exophthalmos, myopathy, and a palpable thyroid constitute the classic syndrome. Laboratory tests such as basal metabolic rate and protein-bound iodine confirm the diagnosis.

(*See also* Endocrine Disorders; Organic Brain Syndrome)

HYPOCHONDRIASIS

Clients are preoccupied with the fear or belief that they have a serious disease, which on physical evaluation is not present. The unrealistic fear or belief persists despite reassurance and causes impairment in social or occupational functioning.

(*See also* Somatoform Disorder)

HYPOGLYCEMIA

An alteration in endocrine functioning which produces both physical and mental symptoms.

Physical symptoms:

Tremor

Light-headedness

Sweating

Hunger

Nausea

Pallor

Tachycardia

Hypertension

Mental Symptoms:

Anxiety

Fugue

Unusual behavior

Confusion

Apathy

Psychomotor agitation or retardation

Depression

Delusions

168

Hallucinations

Convulsions

Coma

(*See also* Endocrine Disorders; Organic Brain Syndrome)

HYPOMANIC

(*See* Manic Behavior)

HYPOTHYROIDISM

The decreased thyroid functioning of myxedema may also alter mental status. Usually the myxedematous client shows slow emotional responses, impaired memory, and slow calculation ability. In severe cases a dementia may develop. Physical changes classically include: thickened, dry skin; coarse, sparse hair; hoarse voice; cold intolerance; bradycardia; edema; hyporeflexia; and deafness. Treatment involves thyroid hormone replacement.

(*See also* Endocrine Disorders; Organic Brain Syndrome)

INTENSIVE CARE UNIT PSYCHOSIS

Developed by clients in intensive care units. This diagnosis is not exact and may refer to any combination of the following: depression, withdrawal, anxiety, hallucinations, delusions, paranoia, and delirium.

The stresses on such a client can be divided into two categories:

Environmental

Sensory overload from constant noise, lights, unfamiliar treatments

Sensory deprivation from immobility, restraints, bandages

Lack of familiar orienting cues such as clocks, calendars, windows, meals, radio, television

Close proximity to other clients who are also very ill

Constant attendance by physicians, nurses, technicians

Lack of personal belongings

Psychologic

Fear of mutilation or death

Little or no understanding of medical jargon or procedures

Separation from family and friends

Separation from familiar environment

Depersonalization and physical exposure

Powerlessness

Pain

Inability to release tension in accustomed fashion

Physiologic stressors

Metabolic changes

Decreased cardiac output

Neurologic status

Fever

Electrolyte imbalance

Drugs

Pain

Length of time spent on pump or under anesthesia

Sleep deprivation

Nursing Intervention

- Elimination of stressors themselves if possible: addition of color and pictures, arrangement of beds for maximum privacy, decreased lighting at night.
- Clients and their families should be adequately prepared if circumstances permit; clients who know what to expect are less frightened by the strangeness of the unit.
- Clients should be provided with consistent nursing personnel. This will diminish the depersonalization and isolation that always occurs to some degree in an intensive care unit.
- Family members can be encouraged to visit as situation permits.
- Needs and frustration of the staff must be attended to; nursing staff should identify ways in which they can support one another.

ID

A psychoanalytic construct: A completely unorganized reservoir of energy derived from a person's drives and instincts.

IDEAS OF REFERENCE

A state in which a person believes that certain events, situations, or interactions are directly related to him or her.

(*See also* Mental Status Examination)

IDENTIFICATION

A defense mechanism in which a person incorporates the mental picture of an object and then patterns the self after that object. Identification is the wish to be like another person and to assume the characteristics of that person's personality. It is unconscious and in this way differs from imitation, which is the conscious copying of another person's qualities.

(*See also* Defense Mechanisms)

IDIOPATHIC SPONTANEOUS HYPOGLYCEMIA

This syndrome is often mistaken for a purely functional psychiatric condition. Idiopathic spontaneous hypoglycemia is hereditary and not necessarily related to stress. A client can experience marked changes in behavior and mood and appear acutely intoxicated as the blood sugar falls below 60 mg/dl. Carbohydrate ingestion rapidly relieves the symptoms.

(*See also* Organic Brain Syndrome)

ILLUSION

Misperceptions and misinterpretations of externally real stimuli. Visual and auditory illusions are much more common than tactile, olfactory, and gustatory illusions.

(*See also* Mental Status Examination; Psychotic Disorders)

IMMEDIACY

A communication skill in which the nurse responds to what is happening between the client and the nurse in the here-and-now.

(*See also* Appendix **C**, Skills That Foster Effective Communication)

IMPARTING INFORMATION

A communication skill in which the nurse makes statements that give needed data to the client and therefore encourage further clarification based on additional input.

(*See also* Appendix **C**, Skills That Foster Effective Communication)

IMPULSIVE BEHAVIOR

Behavior that appears to be unpredictable and unmotivated by observable events, situations, or interactions. The individual behaving impulsively is unable to exert socially expected controls and may be verbally or physically destructive, aggressive, or violent.

INCORPORATION

A coping defense mechanism in which a person symbolically takes within the self the attributes of another person.

(*See also* Defense Mechanisms)

INHALANTS

Glue, gasoline, and solvents are being increasingly used to attain a state similar to alcohol intoxication.

(*See also* Drug Use; Substance Use Disorders)

INITIAL INTERVIEW

A data collection element useful in mental health work. It has the following purposes:

To establish rapport with client

To obtain pertinent client data

To initiate client assessment

To make practical arrangements for treatment

The initial interview, sometimes called the intake interview, is crucial in that it sets the stage for subsequent therapeutic contact.

The major tasks of the initial interview are to:

1. Establish rapport and convey an active willingness to address client's suffering
2. Collect pertinent data, including
   a. Presenting problem

      History

      Development

      Manifestations

      Effect on psychosocial functioning
   b. Event causing client to seek services at this time
   c. Other problems in client's current life situation
   d. Psychosocial functioning and development

      Family constellation

      Physical health status

      History of previous emotional difficulties

      History of any therapy

      History of drug use/abuse

      Coping skills and methods of resolving conflict
   e. Present level of motivation
   f. Identifying characteristics

    Name

    Age

    Sex

    Address

    Telephone number

    Marital status

    Occupation

    Employment record

    Cultural and ethnic origins

3. Initiate client assessment
4. Address any initial client resistances
5. Make practical arrangements for treatment

INSANITY
An obsolete medical term for psychosis or mental illness. It continues to be used in legal terminology.

INSIGHT
The ability to understand one's own motives, psychodynamics, and behavior.

INSULIN THERAPY
A treatment for schizophrenia, introduced by Manfred Sakel, now no longer used in most psychiatric hospitals. It consists of the production of coma, with or without convulsions, through the intramuscular administration of insulin.

INTELLECTUALIZATION
A defense mechanism in which intellectual processes are overused to avoid closeness or affective experience and expression. It is closely related to rationalization.

    Intellectualization may inhibit therapeutic work in

two ways: (1) the client may consistently seek explanations and reasons in order to avoid actual behavioral change, and (2) the client may present an always reasonable self and refuse to develop an understanding of emotions.

(*See also* Defense Mechanisms)

INTELLIGENCE TESTS
Instruments designed to measure intelligence. They may provide useful information, particularly in evaluating the presence and degree of mental retardation. Commonly used intelligence tests include the Stanford-Binet test, the Wechsler Adult Intelligence Scale, and the Wechsler Intelligence Scale for Children.

INTERACTION PROCESS ANALYSIS (IPA)
A verbatim and progressive recording of the verbal and nonverbal interactions between client and nurse within a given period of time.

INTROJECTION
A defense or coping mechanism in which one individual accepts another's values and opinions as his or her own.

(*See also* Defense Mechanisms)

INVOLUNTARY COMMITMENT
The legal process by which a person is confined, without consent, to a mental hospital. There are three categories: (1) emergency, (2) temporary or observational, and (3) extended or indeterminate. Criteria vary from state to state.

(*See also* Legal Aspects)

INVOLUTIONAL PSYCHOSIS

Pre-DSM-III medical model diagnostic term for a disorder commonly characterized by insomnia, anxiety, depression, and sometimes paranoid ideas. It is generally first seen in individuals over 45 years of age with no history of previous mental disorder, and it may be associated with menopause in women and climacteric in men.

ISOLATION

An ego defense mechanism that protects a person from experiencing anxiety by separating feelings and impulses from ideas and pushing them out of consciousness. When isolation is completely successful, both feelings and ideas are repressed. When isolation is less complete, the person is aware of an impulse without realizing its significance.

(*See also* Defense Mechanisms)

J

JACOB-CRUTZFELDT DISEASE
A type of presenile dementia that may be caused by a slowly developing viral invasion of the pyramidal and extrapyramidal tracts. Onset can occur in the third decade of life. The dementia is characterized by memory loss, reduced intellectual functioning, speech difficulties, deterioration of social appropriateness, and perceptual problems such as blindness and hallucinations. The neurologic changes are so-called "long tract" signs, such as muscle wasting, hyperreflexia, clonus, and positive Babinski's reflex.

(*See also* Organic Brain Syndrome)

JUDGMENT
The capacity to anticipate the consequences of one's behavior and to eliminate behaviors that are ineffective. It involves the ability to behave appropriately in terms of external reality and is closely linked with reality testing.

(*See also* Mental Status Examination)

KORSAKOFF'S SYNDROME

Korsakoff's syndrome is a condition resulting from prolonged use of alcohol. Its direct cause is a deficiency of the vitamin thiamine due to poor dietary habits associated with chronic alcoholism. The classical signs of Korsakoff's syndrome are global memory loss and striking confabulation. In DSM III, Korsakoff's syndrome is called "alcohol-induced amnestic disorder."

(*See also* Organic Brain Syndrome)

L

LAS

(*See* Local Adaptation Syndrome)

LATENT

Unconscious or unrevealed; below the surface but potentially able to achieve expression.

LEARNED HELPLESSNESS

Characterized by attempts to establish and maintain contact by adopting a helpless, powerless stance.

Nursing Interventions

- Set clear, firm, and consistent limits on various forms of excessive dependency.
- Avoid retaliatory actions, including withdrawal.
- Emphasize client's determination of and accountability for personal feelings, thoughts, and behaviors.
- Avoid making decisions about, guiding, or otherwise assuming responsibility for client's behavior.
- Give positive reinforcement for development of more independent, growth-facilitating behaviors over time.

LEGAL ASPECTS

Each state has statutes spelling out procedures for admission to and discharge from mental hospitals. Some states also have statutes on the medical and legal rights of individuals once they are in the hospital.

There are two major categories of hospitalization:

1. *Voluntary.* Admission comes about by written

application for admission by the prospective client, or by someone acting in his behalf (parent or guardian). Client has a right to demand and obtain release. However, most states have a "grace period" during which client agrees to give notice—usually in writing—of intention to leave. During this time physician and staff need to examine client to make a decision about changing his status to involuntary.

2. *Involuntary.* Most states provide for more than one involuntary hospitalization procedure. Involuntary hospitalization comes about when a designated body such as a court, administrative tribunal, or a required number of physicians find that the prospective client's mental state meets the statutory criteria for involuntary admission. This varies from state to state. Most states allow for involuntary hospitalization if the client is dangerous to himself or others. Three types of involuntary hospitalization are available in most states.

   a. *Emergency.* A temporary measure with short-term goals. Deals with prevention of behavior likely to create a "clear and present" danger to the client or others

   b. *Temporary or observational.* Commitment of an allegedly mentally deranged individual for a specified period of time to allow for adequate observation so that a diagnosis can be made and treatment instituted

   c. *Extended or indeterminate.* Can come about through either judicial or nonjudicial procedures. In judicial cases, the court may order the patient hospitalized for an extended period (60–180 days) or for an indeterminate time. Nonjudicial procedures for extended involuntary hospitalization include both administrative and medical certification.

TABLE 8. VOLUNTARY AND INVOLUNTARY HOSPITALIZATION

VOLUNTARY ADMISSION

	Informal	Voluntary
Release	Anytime	Usually conditional
Use	Limited	Increasing
Criteria for admission	Client request	Client request

Rights of clients vary from state to state but generally include:

- Provisions for client communication and correspondence
- Restrictions regarding use of mechanical restraints
- Client consent needed for psychosurgery and electroconvulsive therapy
- Periodic review of involuntary clients to protect against spending more time than necessary in hospital

LETHALITY ASSESSMENT

An attempt to predict the likelihood of suicide to guide the helping person's behavior. It may be used to decide whether to hospitalize a suicidal person and what alternatives the person has other than suicide.

Hoff* suggests that an adequate lethality assessment includes:

1. *Suicide plan.* Does person have suicidal ideas? Is the person considering a highly lethal method, or one of low lethality? Are the means for carrying out

*Hoff, L.A. 1984: *People in Crisis: Understanding and Helping,* 2e. Menlo Park, Calif.: Addison-Wesley Publishing Co., p. 186.

INVOLUNTARY ADMISSION

Emergency	Temporary	Extended
Average after 5–10 days	After from 72 hours–60 days	After from 60–180 days or after an indeterminate time
Increasing	Increasing	Decreasing
Usually client dangerousness	Client dangerousness and/or need of care and treatment	Client dangerousness and/or need of care and treatment

suicide available—that is, does the person have access to a gun, pills, ammunition? Has a specific plan been worked out?

2. *History of suicide attempts.* Has the person attempted suicide before? Is the method the same, or is it more or less lethal? What was the outcome of the previous suicide attempt? Was the person rescued accidentally? Has the person been hospitalized for attempting suicide in the past?

3. *Resources and communication with significant others.* What are the person's internal and external resources? Is the person alienated from others?

4. *Age, sex, and race.*

5. *Recent loss.*

6. *Physical illness.*

7. *Drinking and drug abuse.*

8. *Isolation.* Is the person physically alone or emotionally isolated? Are significant others rejecting? Do others fail to approve of the person's role performance?

9. *Unexplained change in behavior.* Change in behavior from careful to careless or impulsive may indicate suicide risk.

10. *Depression.* A significant number of suicide victims are depressed.
11. *Social factors.* A broken home, delinquency and truancy, family discord, unemployment, forced retirement, or a move to another residence may increase a person's risk of suicide.
12. *Mental illness.* If a person's hallucinations command him or her to commit suicide, the risk of suicide is increased. However, it is erroneous to believe that only mentally ill persons commit suicide. Persons with disintegrative life patterns should be assessed according to the other criteria.

A person who fits the first three criteria above is a high suicide risk regardless of other factors, although the others do increase the risk.

An accurate lethality assessment can be used to determine whether to hospitalize a suicidal person and what alternatives the person has other than suicide. It serves as a guide for the intervener.

Lethality of Suicide Methods*:

LOW LETHALITY METHODS	HIGH LETHALITY METHODS
Wrist cutting	Gun
House gas	Jumping
Nonprescription drugs excluding acetylsalicylic acid (aspirin) and acetominophen (Tylenol)	Hanging
	Drowning
	Carbon monoxide poisoning
Tranquilizers	Barbiturates or other prescribed sleeping pills

LOW LETHALITY METHODS	HIGH LETHALITY METHODS
	Aspirin and Tylenol (high doses)
	Car crash
	Exposure to extreme cold

*Adapted from Hoff, L.A. 1984. *People in Crisis: Understanding and Helping.* 2nd ed. Menlo Park, Calif.: Addison-Wesley Publishing Co., p. 186.

(*See also* Suicide)

LINKING
A communication skill in which the nurse responds to the client in a way that ties together two events, experiences, feelings, or persons. It may be useful in connecting the past with current behaviors.

(*See also* Appendix **C**, Skills That Foster Effective Communication)

LITHIUM THERAPY
The treatment of manic or hypomanic states with lithium salts.

(*See also* Appendix **B**, Lithium)

LOCAL ADAPTATION SYNDROME (LAS)
The manifestation of stress in a limited part of the body (for example, the body tissues that are directly subjected to stress in an infected wound).

LOOSENESS OF ASSOCIATION

A phenomenon commonly observed in schizophrenic disorders whereby an apparently unrelated experience or idea reminds a person of some other experience or idea.

(*See also* Mental Status Examination; Psychotic Disorders)

MAGICAL THINKING

A regression to a phase of development when one believed that merely thinking about an event could make it happen. Inherent in magical thinking is the idea of omnipotence of thought. Therefore an impulse to commit vile acts is equated by the person with actually doing them.

(*See also* Mental Status Examination; Psychotic Disorders)

MANIC BEHAVIOR

Characterized by elevated, expansive, or irritable mood and some of the following:

1. Decreased need for sleep
2. More energy than usual
3. Inflated self-esteem
4. Increased productivity
5. Extreme gregariousness
6. Hypersexuality
7. Involvement in activities without concern for the consequences
8. Physical restlessness
9. Unusual talkativeness
10. Exaggeration of past achievements
11. Inappropriate laughing, joking, and running

(*See also* Bipolar Affective Disorder; Lithium in Appendix **B,** Psychotic Disorders)

Nursing Intervention

■ *Decrease environmental stimulation.* Hyperactivity

among manic clients can become life threatening. Keep noise level down, lighting low, and surroundings as simple and calm as possible. Also remove hazardous objects and substances.

- *Provide adequate hygiene, nutrition, and rest.* Not unlike depressed clients, manic clients may need help in meeting their basic human needs. High-calorie foods and drinks are recommended. A place to take short but frequent naps may encourage adequate rest. Client may need reminders to wash or bathe.

- *Provide activities that decrease energy and tension.* Such activities may include vigorous housekeeping chores, jogging, and exercise.

- *Monitor medication.* Most manic clients are treated with lithium carbonate. Assess effects of this medication and identify side and toxic effects. However, major emphasis should be directed toward teaching clients on lithium therapy about their treatment. Discuss the fact that the medication must be taken regularly and perhaps for life. Clients should be taught to recognize symptoms of lithium toxicity and to notify their physician immediately if any symptoms appear. Such symptoms include:

    A feeling of sluggishness

    Lethargy

    A fine tremor or muscle twitching

    Ataxia

If untreated these early toxic symptoms can progress to semiconsciousness and coma. Seizures can also occur in association with electrolyte changes. Thus client must be aware of any other conditions that alter electrolyte balance like vomiting, diarrhea, or excessive perspiration.

MANIC DEPRESSIVE DISORDER

Older diagnostic term for a group of disintegrative reactions whose chief characteristic is mood swings, ranging from profound depression to acute mania, with periods of relative normality between psychotic episodes. Called Bipolar Affective Disorder in DSM III.

(See also Bipolar Affective Disorder)

MANIPULATION

A behavior pattern characterized by attempts to exploit, or actual exploitation of, interpersonal contact. Manipulation occurs in one-to-one relationship work when the client maneuvers to have the therapist meet the client's immediate needs. Manipulative methods may be exhibitionistic, seductive, masochistic, or immature in nature. When manipulation is successful, the client's experience is not a constructive one. Nurses who allow themselves to be manipulated reinforce the client's use of the existing dysfunctional behavior pattern and engage in a mutually maladaptive relationship.

The primary intervention strategy in a manipulative behavior pattern is to provide clear, firm, and consistent expectations in which the therapeutic interests of the client are foremost.

MEDICATIONS

(See Appendix **B:** Psychotropic Medications)

MEGAVITAMIN THERAPY

(See Orthomolecular Medicine)

MENTAL DISORDER

According to DSM III, a behavioral or psychologic pattern that occurs in an individual and is associated with either a painful symptom (distress) or impairment in important areas of functioning (disability).

MENTAL HEALTH/HUMAN SERVICE WORKER

The newest addition to the roster of persons on the psychiatric team. May be "indigenous nonprofessionals" or graduates of 2-year associate degree programs. They bridge the gap between middle-class professionals and clients from lower socioeconomic or otherwise disadvantaged populations.

MENTAL MECHANISMS

(See Defense Mechanisms)

MENTAL RETARDATION

A developmental disability resulting in subnormal intellectual functioning that may be evident at birth or may develop during childhood. Learning, social adjustment, and maturation are impaired, and emotional disturbance may be present.

Assessment

In general, a retarded person has difficulty learning. The more complex the learning task, the more evident the retarded person's limitations. Cognitive processes in which deficits or inabilities may account for difficulties in learning include:

- Arousal of attention
- Direction of attention
- Maintenance of attention
- Sensation

- Perception
- Inhibition of already learned responses
- Abstraction
- Generalization

Retardation may result from disordered brain functioning secondary to structural or metabolic disease or due to a failure to develop physiologic maturity because of genetic abnormality, disease, or profound lack of stimulation.

PROBLEMS ENCOUNTERED BY THE RETARDED

1. High vulnerability to emotional instability because of both constitutional deficiencies and interpersonal input from family and peers
2. Problematic behavioral manifestations such as:
   a. Irritability
   b. Hypersensitivity to environmental stimuli
   c. Tendency to motoric hyperactivity
   d. Restlessness
   e. Short attention span
   f. Poor impulse control
   g. Tendency to act out
3. Difficulty forming and maintaining meaningful human relationships
4. Rejection by family based on parents' anxiety, fear, anger, insecurity, guilt, or threats to self-esteem, or overprotection by family to compensate for feelings of rejection or out of a heightened sense of compassion
5. High percentage of diagnoses of adjustment disorders, depressive disorders, organic brain syndromes, and certain psychotic disorders
6. Pathologic personality profile of the retarded person with moderate to severe emotional dysfunction is:

(Text continues on page 195)

TABLE 9. METABOLIC DISORDERS ASSOCIATED WITH MENTAL RETARDATION

NUTRIENT AFFECTED	EXAMPLE	ESSENTIAL DEFECT	CLINICAL FEATURES	TREATMENT
Amino acid (protein)	Phenylketonuria	Decreased phenylalanine hydroxylase	Blond hair, blue eyes, small size, light complexion, coarse features, small head, hyperactivity, autism	Decrease dietary phenylalanine
	Maple syrup urine disease	Decreased amino acid decarboxylase	Onset at 1 week of age, decerebrate rigidity, seizures, respiratory difficulties, hypoglycemia	Decrease dietary amino acids
Lipid (fat)	Tay-Sachs disease	Decreased hexoaminodase A	Onset at 4–8 months of age, hypotonus, apathy, spasticity, primitive reflexes, cherry spot retina, convulsions	None

	Gaucher's disease	Decreased glucocerebrosidase	Onset in infancy or before 10 years, hepatosplenomegaly, abdominal and cranial enlargement, hypotonia, opisthotonos	None
Carbohydrate (starch)	Galactosemia	Decreased galactose-1-phosphate uridyltransferase	Onset 1 week after birth, jaundice, vomiting, diarrhea, failure to thrive, hepatomegaly, cataracts	Decrease dietary galactose
	Glycogen storage disease	Absent glycogen metabolism	Onset in neonatal period, hepatomegaly, failure to thrive, acidosis, hypoglycemic convulsions	Symptomatic

(Continued)

193

TABLE 9. METABOLIC DISORDERS ASSOCIATED WITH MENTAL RETARDATION (Continued)

NUTRIENT AFFECTS	EXAMPLE	ESSENTIAL DEFECT	CLINICAL FEATURES	TREATMENT
Miscellaneous	Idiopathic hyper-calcemia	Hypersensitivity to vitamin D	Irritability, elfin facies, short stature, hypotonia, hypertension, strabismus, nephrocalcinosis	Cortisone
	Wilson's disease	Decreased copper ceruloplasmin	Onset in juvenile or adult, cirrhosis, pseudobulbar palsy, wing-flapping, Kayser-Fleischer ring	Penicillamine, dimercaprol
	Hurler's syndrome	Increased dermatan sulfate or increased heparan sulfate	Bone and skull malformations, hepatosplenomegaly, dwarfism, hypertelorism	None

a. Autism
b. Repetition
c. Inflexibility
d. Passivity
e. Immaturity
f. Deficiency in ego function

Nursing Intervention

Simplicity, patience, and support are hallmarks of a successful approach in treating the retarded child psychotherapeutically.

- Provide very concrete, reality-oriented, and pleasure-oriented experiences.
- Create an accepting and affectionate atmosphere.
- Be willing to try to meet considerable dependency needs.
- Foster a sense of self-worth or value in the individual to counteract the forces that induce feelings of rejection and worthlessness.

Treatment consists of:

- *Group therapy.* May be a potentially reinforcing experience for retarded adolescents
- *Behavior modification.* Can be used when behavioral difficulties predominate
- *Family intervention.* Recommended from the birth of a retarded person to assist parents in dealing with shock and sense of loss. Treatment team should be aware that emotional distress occurs for parents as the result of stress and should be alert for signs of developing problems.

Countertransference may result from feelings of frustration and anger. The key to adoptive response in nurse, client, and family is the maintenance of a reasonable degree of hopefulness by reinforcement of the retarded person's inherent value.

MENTAL STATUS EXAMINATION

Usually a standardized procedure with the primary purpose of gathering data to determine etiology, diagnosis, prognosis, and treatment. The mental status examiner generally seeks the following information,* though not necessarily in the sequence presented here:

1. *General behavior and appearance.* A complete and accurate description of the client's physical characteristics, apparent age, manner of dress, use of cosmetics, personal hygiene, and responses to the examiner. Postures, gait, gestures, facial expressions, and mannerisms are included in the descriptions. The examiner also notes the client's general activity level.

   A 35-year-old, white male, dressed in torn, disheveled jeans. Presented a blank facial expression, slouched posture, shuffling gait, generally low-activity level, and sullen behavior.

2. *Characteristics of talk.* The form, rather than the content, of the client's speech. The speech is described in terms of loudness, flow, speed, quantity, level of coherence, and logic. A sample of the client's conversation with the examiner may be included. The following patterns, if present, should be particularly noted.

   a. *Mutism.* No verbal response from the client despite indications that he or she is aware of the examiner's questions.

   b. *Circumstantiality.* Cumbersome and convoluted detail volunteered by the client but unnecessary to answer the interviewer's questions.

   c. *Perseveration.* A pattern of repeating the same

*Reprinted with permission of Sandoz Pharmaceuticals, Division of Sandoz, Inc. From S.M. Small, *Outline for Psychiatric Examination,* 1980.

words or movements despite apparent efforts to make a new response.

d. *Flight of ideas.* Rapid, overly productive responses to questions that seem related only by chance associations between one sentence fragment and another. Associated with flight of ideas might be rhyming, clang associations, punning, and evidence of distractibility.

e. *Blocking.* A pattern of sudden silence in the stream of conversation for no obvious reason but often thought to be associated with intrusion on the client of delusional thoughts or hallucinations.

3. *Emotional state.* The person's mood or affective reaction. Both subjective and objective data are included. Subjective data are obtained through the use of nonleading questions such as: "How are you feeling?" If the client replies by using such general terms as "nervous," he or she should be asked to describe how the nervousness shows itself and its effect, since such words may mean different things to different individuals. The examiner should observe objective signs such as facial expression, motor behavior, and the presence of tears, flushing, sweating, tachycardia, tremors, respiratory irregularities, states of excitement, fear, and depression. Much valuable information may be obtained by noting the relationship between the client and the examiner. Attitudes of hostility, suspiciousness or flirtatiousness, a desire for bodily contact, or outspoken criticisms should be noted.

The psychiatric client is apt to have a persistent emotional trend based on a particular emotional disorder such as depression. If this is true, further inquiry should attempt to reveal the intensity and persistence of this reaction.

It is desirable to record a verbatim reply to questions concerning the client's mood. The relationship between mood and the content of thought is particularly significant. There may be a wide divergence between what the client says or does and his emotional state as expressed by attitudes or facial expressions.

Note whether intense emotional responses accompany discussion of specific topics. *Shallowness* or *flattening of the affect* is indicated by an insufficiently intense emotional display in association with ideas or situations that ordinarily would call for a more adequate response. *Dissociation or disharmony* is often indicated by an inappropriate emotional response, such as smiling or silly behavior, when the attitude should be one of concern, anxiety, or sadness.

Evaluation of emotional reactions may be even more difficult because some clients may use *simulation* or *play-acting*. Clients who are trying to cover up a deep depression may feign cheerfulness and good spirits. The reverse may also be true.

The client's emotional reactions may be constant or may fluctuate during the examination. Try to specify the ease or readiness with which such changes occur in response to pleasant or unpleasant stimuli. Use such terms as the following to indicate intensity of response:

Composed, complacent, frank, friendly; playful, teasing, silly, cheerful, boastful, elated, grandiose, ecstatic

Tense, worried, anxious, pessimistic, sad, perplexed, bewildered, gloomy, depressed, frightened

Aloof, superior, disdainful, distant, defensive, suspicious

Irritable, resentful, hostile, sarcastic, angry, furious

Indifferent, resigned, apathetic, dull, affectless

The relationship of affect to content should be noted in terms of the influence of content on affect and disharmony between affect and content or thought. Constancy and change in the emotional state should be noted.

4. *Special preoccupations and experiences.* Delusions, illusions, hallucinations, depersonalizations, obsessions or compulsions, phobias, fantasies, and daydreams. These data may be elicited by asking the client questions, such as "Do you have any difficulties you complain of?" or "Have you been troubled or ill in any way?"

If the patient has delusions of being the object of environmental attention, some of the following questions might reveal them: "Do people like you?" "Have you ever been watched or spied upon or singled out for special attention?" "Do others have it in for you?"

Delusions of *alien control* (passivity) are feelings of being controlled or guided by external forces. If these delusions are suspected, ask the client such questions as "Do you ever feel your thoughts or actions are under any outside influences or control?" "Is your mind controlled by thought waves, electricity, or radio waves?" "Are you able to influence others, to read their minds, or to put thoughts in their minds?"

Nihilistic delusions are those in which the client more or less completely denies reality and existence. The client states that nothing exists, or everything is lost. He or she may say such things as "I have no head, no stomach," "I cannot die," or "I will live to eternity."

Delusions of *self-deprecation* are often seen in connection with severe depressions. The client describes feelings of unworthiness, sinfulness, ugliness, or emitting obnoxious odors.

Delusions of *grandeur* are associated with elated states, such as great wealth, strength, power, sexual potency, or identification with a famous person—even God.

Somatic delusions are focused on having cancer, obstructed bowels, leprosy, or some horrible disease. This is to be distinguished from a preoccupation with normal visceral, or peripheral sensations.

Hallucinations are false sensory impressions without any external basis in fact. Try to elicit the clearness of the projection to the outside world (for instance, whether the client hears voices from outside or inside his or her head, the clarity and distinctness of the perception, and the intensity). Be tactful in approaching the client for evidences of hallucinatory phenomena unless he or she is obviously hallucinating.

Obsessions are insistent thoughts recognized as arising from the self usually regarded by the client as absurd and relatively meaningless, yet they persist despite endeavors to get rid of them.

Compulsions are repetitive acts performed through some inner need or drive and are supposed to arrive against the subject's wishes and yet produce feelings of tension and anxiety if omitted.

Fantasies and *daydreams* are preoccupations that are often difficult to elicit from the client. The difficulty may be due to a lack of understanding of what the examiner wants, but the client is often ashamed to talk about them because of their content.

5. *Sensorium* or *orientation*. Orientation in terms of time, place, person, and self to determine the presence of confusion or clouding of consciousness. One may introduce such questions by asking "Have you kept track of the time?" If so, "What is today's date?" If the client says he or she does not know, he or she should be asked to estimate approximately or to guess at an answer. Many clinicians begin the mental status exam with these questions since the validity and reliability of subsequent data require that the client be reasonably oriented.

6. *Memory*. The person's attention span and ability to retain or recall past experiences in both the recent and the remote past. If memory loss exists, the examiner should determine whether it is constant or variable and whether the loss is limited to a certain time period. The examiner should be alert to the client's confabulations or attempts to devise memories to take the place of those he or she cannot recall. It is useful to introduce questions relating to memory by some general statement such as "Has your memory been good?" or "Have you had difficulty remembering telephone numbers or appointments?"

   a. *Recall of remote past experiences*. The person can be asked to review the important chronologic facts of his or her life. The information given can be compared with information obtained from other sources during the history-taking process.

   b. *Recall of recent past experiences*. Such as the events leading to the present seeking of treatment.

   c. *Retention and recall of immediate impressions*. The examiner might ask the client to repeat a name, address, and color immediately and again after 3 to 5 minutes, or to repeat three-digit numbers at a rate of one per second, or to repeat a complicated sentence.

d. *General grasp and recall.* The person might be asked to read a story and then repeat the gist of it with as many details as possible. "The Cowboy Story" is an example suggested for this purpose in a concise guide for conducting a psychiatric examination developed by S.M. Small (1980).

THE COWBOY STORY

A cowboy from Arizona went to San Francisco with his dog, which he left at a friend's while he purchased a new suit of clothes. Dressed in the new suit, he went back to the dog, whistled to him, called him by name, and patted him. The dog would have nothing to do with him in his new hat and coat but gave a mournful howl. Coaxing had no effect, so the cowboy went away and donned his old garments. Then the dog immediately showed his wild joy on seeing his master as he thought he ought to be.

7. *General intellectual level.* A nonstandardized evaluation of intelligence. The examiner looks for the person's ability to use factual knowledge in a comprehensive way.

a. *General grasp of information.* The person may be asked to name the five largest cities of the United States, the last four presidents, or the governor of the state.

b. *Ability to calculate.* Tests of simple multiplication and addition may be given. Another test consists of subtracting from 100 by sevens until the person can go no farther (Serial Seven's).

c. *Reasoning and judgment.* Clients are commonly asked what they might do with $10,000 if it were given to them. Examiners must be particularly careful to correct for their own biases and values in assessing each client's answer.

8. *Abstract thinking.* The distinctions between such abstractions as poverty and misery or idleness and laziness. It is common to ask the client to interpret simple fables or proverbs, such as "Don't cry over spilled milk."

9. *Insight evaluation.* Whether the client recognizes the significance of the present situation, whether the client feels the need of treatment, and the client's own explanation of the symptoms. Often it is helpful to ask the client for suggestions for his or her own treatment.

10. *Summary.* The important psychopathologic findings and a tentative diagnosis. Pertinent facts from the medical history and/or physical examination should be added to the summary.

See Table 10, page 204.

MID-LIFE CRISIS

The set of problems that arises when people discover visible signs that they are aging and become preoccupied with the notion of their own mortality. It frequently occurs between 35 and 45 years of age. It is sometimes called an authenticity crisis.

MILIEU

The social and cultural aspects of an environment that can influence the behavior of the person in it.

MILIEU THERAPY

Treatment that emphasizes appropriate socioenvironmental manipulation for the benefit of the client.

MINNESOTA MULTIPHASIC PERSONALITY INVENTORY

(*See* Psychologic Tests)

(*Text continues on page 208.*)

TABLE 10. DIFFERENTIATION OF MENTAL STATUS EXAMINATION FINDINGS*

	ORGANIC BRAIN SYNDROME		MENTAL RETARDATION
	Acute (Delirium)	Chronic (Dementia)	
Appearance and behavior	Fluctuating impairment of consciousness, restlessness	May show deterioration of personal habits but state of consciousness not clouded	
Mood	Anxiety, fear, lability	Irritability, lability	
Thought processes and perceptions			
Coherence and relevance	May be confused, incoherent	May become confused	
Thought content	May have delusions		

*Source: Adapted from Bates, B. 1974. *A Guide to Physical Examination* Philadelphia, J. B. Lippincott Co., pp. 312-313.

DISINTEGRATIVE LIFE PATTERNS (PSYCHOTIC CONDITIONS)		DISTURBED PERSONAL COPING PATTERNS (AFFECTIVE DISORDERS)
Manic Episode	Schizophrenic Disorders	Depression
Hyperactive, elated, assertive, boisterous, with rapid emphatic speech; may become suddenly angry or argumentative	Variable	Dejected, slowed, slumped, troubled
Elation, sometimes anger and irritability	Blandness, impoverishment or inappropriateness of affect	Depression, hopelessness
Rapid association of ideas that may seem illogical	Often incoherent, disorganized	
May have delusions and feelings of persecution	May have feelings of unreality, depersonalization, persecution, influence and reference; delusions that	May have delusions, often involving guilt, self-depreciation, somatic complaints

(Continued)

TABLE 10. DIFFERENTIATION OF MENTAL STATUS EXAMINATION FINDINGS (Continued)

	ORGANIC BRAIN SYNDROME		MENTAL RETARDATION
	Acute (Delirium)	Chronic (Dementia)	

(Thought processes and perceptions, continued)

Perceptions	May have illusions, hallucinations		
Cognitive functions			
Orientation	May be disoriented	May be disoriented	Depends on severity of deficiency
Attention and concentration	Poor	Poor	Limited
Recent memory	Poor	Poor	May be poor
Remote memory	May become poor	May become poor	May be poor

DISINTEGRATIVE LIFE PATTERNS (PSYCHOTIC CONDITIONS)		DISTURBED PERSONAL COPING PATTERNS (AFFECTIVE DISORDERS)
Manic Episode	Schizophrenic Disorders	Depression
May have illusions, rarely hallucinations	are bizarre and symbolic May have hallucinations and illusions, often bizarre and symbolic	May have illusions, rarely hallucinations
Well-oriented	Usually but not always well-oriented	Well-oriented
Distractable		
	Usually well-preserved but may be difficult to test because of inattentiveness and indifference	
	Usually well-preserved but may be difficult to test because of	

(Continued)

TABLE 10. DIFFERENTIATION OF MENTAL STATUS EXAMINATION FINDINGS (Continued)

	ORGANIC BRAIN SYNDROME		MENTAL RETARDATION
	Acute (Delirium)	Chronic (Dementia)	

(Cognitive functions, continued)

Information	Preserved until late	Preserved until late	Limited
Vocabulary	Preserved until late	Preserved until late	Limited
Abstract reasoning	Concrete	Concrete	Concrete
Judgment	Poor	Poor	May be poor
Perception and coordination	May be poor	May be poor	May be poor

M'NAGHTEN RULES

The legal rules used in most English-speaking courts to determine whether a psychiatrically ill person is responsible for a criminal act he or she committed. They are based mainly on whether the person knew the "nature and quality" of the act and that doing it was "wrong."

(See also Legal Aspects)

DISINTEGRATIVE LIFE PATTERNS (PSYCHOTIC CONDITIONS)		DISTURBED PERSONAL COPING PATTERNS (AFFECTIVE DISORDERS)
Manic Episode	Schizophrenic Disorders	Depression
	inattentiveness and indifference	
	Concrete, may be bizarre	

MONGOLISM

(See Down's Syndrome)

MONOAMINE-OXIDASE INHIBITOR

An agent that inhibits the enzyme monoamine oxidase (MAO), which oxidizes such monoamines as norepinephrine and serotonin. Some MAO inhibitors are highly effective as antidepressants.

(*See also* Appendix **B,** Antidepressant Drugs)

MOURNING

(*See* Grief Work/Grieving)

MULTIPLE PERSONALITY

A dissociative pattern in which the person is dominated by two or more distinct personalities, each of which determines the person's behavior and attitudes during the period that it is uppermost in consciousness.

(*See also* Dissociative Disorders)

MULTIPLE SCLEROSIS

Also known as disseminated sclerosis, this degeneration of cerebral tissue is characterized by diffuse neurologic symptoms, due to demyelination of nerve fibers in many areas of the nervous system. The symptoms tend to wax and wane rather than progress steadily. It is rare for frank psychosis, delirium, or dementia to occur, but emotional instability is commonly encountered and may well have an organic component. There is no treatment for the disease itself, only for its symptoms.

N

NARCISSISTIC PERSONALITY DISORDER

(*See* Personality Disorder)

NARCOTHERAPY

The use of intravenous barbiturates and stimulants to facilitate a client's expression of highly charged feelings. Also called sodium amytal interview and "truth serum." This is a two-step process:

1. *Emotional catharsis.* The mere reliving or re-experiencing of emotions associated with a traumatic event, which have been submerged deep in the unconscious, has a beneficial effect.
2. *Narcosynthesis.* Consists of interpretations or other psychotherapeutic interventions by the therapist. These are more easily accepted by a client under the drug's influence and thus perhaps more available for insight (client is less resistant).

   The major danger in the treatment is that of laryngospasm secondary to intravenous barbiturates.

NEOLOGISM

A private, unshared meaning of a word or term. Neologisms are frequently characteristic of the language of schizophrenic individuals. The person labeled schizophrenic may use language in an idiosyncratic way. Such a person is unaware that this use of language is not shared with others. He or she expects to be understood by them and may become upset when this does not occur.

(*See also* Mental Status Examination; Psychotic Disorders)

NEOPLASMS

Intracranial tumors of any variety can produce mental changes ranging from exaggeration of preexisting personality traits to dementia or delusions. Frequently, the type of mental symptom helps to locate the tumor in the brain. For example, apathy or the progressive loss of intellectual functions suggests frontal lobe pathology, while memory loss, fear, depersonalization, *déjà vu* (paramnesia), derealization, temper outbursts, and olfactory hallucinations are indicative of a temporal lobe lesion. Body image changes, ignoring part of the body, loss of sense of direction, and visual hallucinations usually indicate a parietal lobe problem. Flashing lights correlate with occipital tumors. Diagnostic physical findings usually relate to each location as well after tumors reach significant size. Treatment is surgical.

(*See also* Organic Brain Syndrome)

NEUROLOGIC ASSESSMENT

(*See* Physiologic and Neurologic Assessment)

NEUROFIBROMATOSIS

This condition, also known as von Recklinghausen's disease, affects the skin and the central nervous system. It is inherited through dominant genes. Although there are gross neurologic and dermatologic findings, such as nodules, polyps, nevi, *café au lait* spots, sensory loss, and nerve deafness, the first signs may be altered behavior: hyperirritability, erratic behavior of abrupt onset, or even florid psychosis. The condition usually leads to increased intracranial pressure and seizures.

(*See also* Organic Brain Syndrome)

NEUROSIS

A pre-DSM-III mental disorder characterized by anxiety. In DSM III, the neurotic disorders are included in affective, anxiety, somatoform, dissociative, and psychosexual disorder categories.

(*See* Neurotic Disorders)

NEUROTIC DISORDERS

A category of behavior traditionally called psychoneurosis in psychiatric terminology. It is characterized by loss of ability to make choices, conflict, repetition, rigidity, ineffective solutions, alienation, feelings of being troubled and distressed, and secondary gain.

NIACIN THERAPY

(*See* Orthomolecular Medicine)

NICOTINE

Central nervous system stimulant that acts both as a stimulant and a depressant. It is a highly toxic drug: 60 mg constitutes a lethal dose. Nicotine has been related to lung cancer, coronary artery disease, and emphysema.

NIHILISTIC DELUSION

(*See* Delusion)

NONCOMPLIANCE

Self-destructive behavior that interferes with the therapeutic plan. There is always a reason for noncompliance, although neither the nurse nor the patient may initially understand the dynamics involved. Many nurses respond to such clients with anger and impatience, which serves only to increase the distance between patient and nurse. It is admittedly very difficult to watch self-destructive behavior that thwarts what one believes to be the correct therapeutic route. The nurse can reach an understanding of the patient's behavior only through careful thought and observation.

In general, the factors that contribute to noncompliance can be summarized as follows:

- *Psychologic.* Lack of knowledge; clients' attitudes, beliefs, and values; denial of illness and other defense mechanisms; personality type (rigid, defensive, etc.), and very low or very high anxiety levels
- *Environmental and social.* Lack of support system; other problems that distract from health care; and finances, transportation, and housing
- *Characteristics of the regimen.* Demands too much change from client; not enough benefit realized; too difficult, complicated; distressing side effects; leads to social isolation and stigma
- *Properties of the provider-patient relationship.* Faulty communication; client perceives provider as cold, uncaring, authoritative; client feels discounted and treated like an "object"; both parties engage in struggle for control

Nursing Intervention

The "contract" approach can deal with noncompliance as well as prevent its occurrence. A contract is a mutual verbal or written agreement between client and nurse about their expectations of each other. It makes clear that they are equal partners with certain responsibilities toward established common goals.

The contract makes expectations, goals and responsibilities explicit.

NONCONVULSIVE ELECTRICAL STIMULATION THERAPY

A new approach has been derived from conventional electroconvulsive therapy (ECT). It is well known that subconvulsive stimuli during ECT are associated with poor therapeutic response. Proponents of nonconvulsive treatment agree that this is true for clients for whom standard ECT is indicated. They argue, however, that a large group of clients for whom ECT is not indicated are responsive to nonconvulsive electrical stimulation. These include clients suffering from behaviors traditionally labeled anxiety neurosis, phobic neurosis, depressive neurosis, and personality disorders. As yet there are no controlled studies of this method.

NURSING CARE PLAN

A means of providing nursing personnel with information about the needs and therapeutic strategy for each client. When source-oriented recording methods are used, it may provide an ongoing, up-to-date record of goal-directed individual nursing care. When problem-oriented recording methods are used, the nursing plan may be an outgrowth of the record.

An effective nursing care plan:

- Identifies priorities of care
- States realistic goals in measurable terms with an expected date of accomplishment
- Is based on identifiable psychotherapeutic principles
- Indicates which client needs are the primary responsibility of the psychiatric nurse and which

will be referred to others with appropriate expertise

■ Reflects mutual goal setting and shared responsibility for goal attainment at the level of client's abilities

■ Forms basis for client care activities done by others under nurse's supervision

(*See also* Problem-Oriented Recording)

NURSING DIAGNOSIS

The conceptualization of a client's need, problem, or situation from the unique perspective of the theoretic constructs in the discipline of nursing.

CATEGORIES OF NURSING DIAGNOSES FOR PSYCHIATRIC CLIENTS

1. Self-care limitations or impaired functioning with general etiologies (such as mental and emotional distress), deficits in the ways significant systems are functioning, and internal psychic or developmental issues relevant to health

2. Emotional stress or crisis components of illness, pain, self-concept changes, and life process changes

3. Emotional problems related to daily experiences such as anxiety, aggression, loss, loneliness, and grief

4. Physical symptoms, such as altered intestinal functioning or anorexia, which occur simultaneously with altered psychic functioning

5. Alterations in thinking, perceiving, symbolizing, communication, and decision-making abilities

6. Behaviors and mental states that indicate client is a danger to self or others or is gravely disabled

NURSING HISTORY

The foremost method of collecting data from a primary source (the client). Differs from medical or psychiatric histories in that it focuses on client's perception and explanation related to illness, hospitalization and care.

NURSING PROCESS
The conscious systematic set of cognitive behavioral steps that comprise the clinical act in nursing practice.

O

OBESITY
Weight gain resulting from the intake of foods in amounts exceeding physical needs. Hunger and satiety are under the control of the hypothalmus. This organ is programmed to respond to a wide range of factors including:

Socioeconomic status

Genetic determinants

Developmental considerations

Physical activity

Brain damage

Emotional factors

Many people, obese and normal, tend to overeat when they are emotionally distressed. Obese individuals, however, seem particularly susceptible to frustrations in love relationships. People with weight problems show poor self-control when it comes to eating behavior and a high-response level to social cues, rather than physiologic stimuli to eat. These people frequently have body image disturbances that either help cause or result from their overeating patterns. Many obese individuals have a low self-concept and act out self-critical, self-punitive rituals with overeating, commonly in "binges."

(See also Psychophysiologic Disorder)

OBSESSION
A persistent idea, thought, or impulse that cannot be eliminated from consciousness by logical effort. This

thought is sometimes trivial or ridiculous, often morbid or fearful, and usually distressing and anxiety provoking.

(*See also* Compulsive Personality Disorder)

OPPOSITIONAL DISORDERS
A pattern, for at least 6 months, of disobedient, negativistic behavior.

Assessment

The onset is after 3 years and before 18 years of age. General symptoms include violations of rules, temper tantrums, provocative behavior, argumentativeness, and stubbornness—with no violation of the basic rights of others or of major age-appropriate societal norms or rules. Excessive rebelliousness can include frequent temper tantrums, fighting, destruction of toys and other objects, and consistent oppositional behavior. This should not be confused with the expression of negativism that is normal at around 2 years of age, which is a necessary (although trying) developmental stage. Excessive rebelliousness usually indicates a frightened child. Inconsistency in handling the child, the setting of rigid limits, or the parents' refusal or inability to set limits all can create insecurity and fear in the child.

Nursing Intervention

Offer parent counseling if necessary. When working with the child, be receptive and sympathetic while establishing and maintaining firm limits.

ORGANIC BRAIN SYNDROME
Mental or behavioral changes associated with physiologic processes occurring in the brain. Potentially reversible causes of organic brain syndrome include:

1. Vascular disorders
   a. Hemorrhage
   b. Hypertension
   c. Systemic lupus erythematosus
2. Infectious disorders
   a. Meningoencephalitis
   b. Brain abscess
   c. Tertiary syphilis
3. Traumatic disorders
   a. Hematoma
   b. Communicating hydrocephalus
4. Metabolic disorders
   a. Hepatic failure
   b. Renal failure
   c. Chronic obstructive pulmonary disease
   d. Electrolyte imbalance
   e. Inappropriate antidiuretic hormone
   f. Wilson's disease
5. Poisons
   a. Barbiturates
   b. Heavy metals
6. Endocrine disorders
   a. Thyroid disease
   b. Parathyroid disease
   c. Cushing's disease
   d. Addison's disease
   e. Hypoglycemia
7. Deficiency states
   a. Pernicious anemia
   b. Wernicke-Korsakoff's syndrome

Clinical features of delirium and dementia, two major types of organic brain syndrome:

FEATURE	DELIRIUM	DEMENTIA
Onset	Acute	Either acute or insidious

FEATURE	DELIRIUM	DEMENTIA
Level of consciousness	Clouding with either hyperactivity or somnolence	No clouding
Cognitive impairment	Fluctuating, worse at night	Severe, recent memory impaired first
Disorientation	Present	Absent
Electroencephalogram pattern	Slowing	Unreliable, may be normal
Special characteristics	Disturbance of sleep pattern, hallucinations, delusions, incoherence	Impaired abstract thinking and judgment, evidence of cerebral cortical dysfunction, personality change
Prognosis	Depends on cause	Depends on cause

Certain major physical conditions that lead to organic brain syndrome occur with increased frequency among the elderly population, but the syndromes can complicate illnesses in all age groups.

Assessment

The assessment of organicity is a task relevant to psychological testing. Changes in cognitive functions—alterations in the information processing systems of the brain—are usually interpreted as indicating organicity. Areas of impairment that identify organicity include:

- Attention span
- Concentration
- Language skills
- Memory
- Orientation
- Thinking

    Learning

    Abstraction

    Reasoning

    Concept formation

Organic brain syndromes usually manifest some degree of organicity as part of the clinical picture, but changes in behavior and emotion brought about by cerebral pathology are by no means limited to those commonly described as organicity.

Nursing Intervention

Nurses should be aware of the variables affecting patient response to treatment. These include:

- *Level of sensory input to clients.* Too great or too little sensory input can precipitate further cognitive, perceptual, and affective deterioration.
- *Degree of social isolation experienced by clients.* Clients with organic mental syndromes need contacts with other human beings, especially well-known family members. The contacts may be rather simple and uncomplicated, but they must be familiar and reliable.
- *Unfamiliarity of environment to clients.* Clients need a setting that is readily recognizable. Family members can bridge the gap between hospital and home by regular visiting.
- *Interpersonal network available to clients.* These people, especially, need a loving, reliable, and sup-

portive social network around them. Interventions with family and friends might range from simple explanations about the nature of the illness to suggestions about what might be helpful to full-fledged family therapy.

ORTHOMOLECULAR MEDICINE

An increasingly popular approach to the treatment of schizophrenia, in which large doses of vitamins (ascorbic acid, niacinamide, pyridoxine, and vitamin E) are administered to clients. Also called megavitamin therapy and niacin therapy.

P

PANIC
An acute, intense attack of anxiety associated with extreme personality disorganization.

PANIC DISORDER
A type of disturbed coping pattern characterized by sudden, intense, and discrete periods of extreme fear accompanied by symptoms such as dyspnea, palpitations, chest pain, choking sensations, dizziness, derealization, paresthesias, hot and cold flashes, sweating, faintness, trembling or shaking, and a fear of impending doom.

(See also Anxiety)

PARANOID PERSONALITY DISORDER
A disruptive life style characterized by hypersensitivity, rigidity, suspiciousness, jealous envy, and self-importance. The individual tends to blame others and feel they have a malevolent intent. He or she feels mistreated and misjudged. There may be:

Expectations of trickery or harm

Guardedness or secretiveness

Jealousy

Doubt of others' loyalty

Over concern with hidden motives and special meanings.

Paranoid people avoid surprise by anticipating it. There is also a tendency to be easily slighted, to make mountains out of molehills, and to find it very difficult to relax. Paranoid people construct a subjective world in which facts, accurately enough perceived in themselves, are endowed with a special interpretive significance. The subject matter of their interest has to do with hidden motives, underlying purposes, special meanings, and the like. Projection is the ego defense mechanism in which paranoid people attribute to external figures the motivations, drives, or other feelings that are present in, but intolerable to, themselves.

(*See also* Personality Disorders)

Nursing Intervention

- Re-establish attenuated communication and feedback with the client.
- Diminish the social isolation that reinforces the client's idea that something is wrong.
- Keep verbal and nonverbal messages clear and consistent.
- Avoid engaging in pretexts, trickery, and deception to enlist the client's cooperation.
- Offer a basis for establishing consensual validation of reality without belittling the client's experience of it (for example, it is preferable to state, "I don't interpret things in that way, but I understand from what you've said that you do," than to assert, "You're wrong, it's not that way at all").

The fundamental principle in working effectively with these clients is to convey to them that you do not perceive reality in the same way they do but are willing to listen, learn, and offer feedback about their experiences and concerns. Other guidelines in working with suspicious clients include:

- To foster trust, follow through on commitments made to the client.

- To help minimize anxiety, plan several brief contacts with the client rather than one prolonged contact.
- To decrease fear, provide environmental supports such as a night light.
- To increase cooperation, respect client's privacy and preferences as much as is reasonable.
- To avoid misinterpretation and enhance trust, be as honest and open with the client as possible.

PARAPHRASING

An activity or communication skill in which the nurse restates what she or he has heard the client communicating. It offers an opportunity to test the nurse's understanding of what the client is attempting to communicate.

(*See also* Appendix **C**, Skills That Foster Effective Communication)

PARATHYROID HYPERFUNCTION

Tumors of the parathyroid, both benign and malignant, and cellular hyperplasia cause excess production of parathyroid hormone. This elevates the blood calcium levels, which lead to manifestations of organic mental syndrome. There may be alterations in mood, such as depression, impairment of intellectual abilities, stupor, or psychosis. Some clients who complain of weakness, irritability, and bone pain may be mistaken as neurotic. Physically there are signs of calcium deposits in the conjunctiva and eyelids, as well as facial palsy, auditory impairment, and possibly hypertension. Treatment may involve surgical removal of tumor.

(*See also* Organic Brain Syndrome)

PARATHYROID HYPOFUNCTION

May result from surgical removal of the parathyroid glands, either for the treatment of hyperfunction or accidentally (for example, in thyroid surgery), from dietary deficiencies of calcium or vitamin D, or from malabsorption in the intestines. In general, hypocalcemia leads to excitable central nervous system states that may manifest themselves as acute delirium, complete with agitation, disorientation, confusion and hallucinations; intellectual deterioration; odd or neurotic behavior; catatonia; or convulsions. Physical examination reveals hair loss, dry skin, deterioration of the teeth, cataracts, and signs of tentany—that is, Trousseau's and Chvostek's signs. Treatment is accomplished by replacing parathormone, giving vitamin D, or giving calcium lactate.

(See also Organic Brain Syndrome)

PARKINSONIAN SYNDROME

A syndrome that may occur after a week or two of antipsychotic medication therapy that bears a striking resemblance to Parkinson's disease. It is characterized by masklike faces, resting tremor, general rigidity of posture with slow voluntary movement, and a shuffling gait. Treatable with an antiparkinsonian agent.

(See also Appendix **B**, Antiparkinsonian Drugs)

PASSIVE-AGGRESSIVE PERSONALITY DISORDER

Characterized by use of passive behavior to express hostility. The behavior includes obstructionism, pouting, procrastination, stubbornness, and intentional inefficiency.

These people appear dependent and lack self-confidence, but their most consistent characteristic is resistance to demands for occupational and social performance expressed indirectly through such maneuvers as dawdling and forgetfulness. These behaviors persist even under circumstances in which more assertive and effective patterns are possible.

(*See also* Personality Disorders)

PELLAGRA
This condition is associated with "the three Ds": dermatitis, diarrhea, and dementia. Its cause is dietary deficiency of nicotinic acid, which can occur in alcoholics or in a population with very poor nutrition. In addition to the classic signs of dementia, symptoms include a swollen tongue, pathologic sucking and grasping reflexes, decreased deep tendon reflexes, rigidity, and pain corresponding to nerve pathways. Treatment is with nicotinic acid.

(*See also* Organic Brain Syndrome)

PERCEPTION
The experience of sensing, interpreting, and comprehending the world; a highly personal and internal act.

(*See also* Mental Status Examination; Psychotic Disorders)

PERSECUTION, DELUSIONS OF
(*See* Delusions)

PERSEVERATION
A pattern of repeating the same words or movements despite apparent efforts to make a new response.

PERSONALITY DISORDERS
In DSM III these include eccentric or odd, dramatic or emotional, and anxious or fearful Axis II disorders.

Although each of the personality disorders has certain unique characteristics, some common properties exist. They include:
1. They are primarily defensive modes of living.
2. They are usually related to some form of arrested behavior development or to overdevelopment of a particular pattern or trait.
3. Problems are expressed through general behavior, rather than through the development of any particular symptoms in response to stress.
4. The behavior that expresses these problems is troubling to others, thus these people usually come into conflict with others, either in their immediate families or in society at large.
5. Disruptive lifestyles become deeply ingrained and are very difficult to modify or change.
6. Most of the behavior is governed by infantile, pleasure-oriented forces, with inadequate control of moral sensitivity (superego) or problem-solving and reality-testing skills (ego functions).
7. The ability to develop meaningful relationships with others and to communicate effectively is seriously impaired.
8. The person rarely recognizes or acknowledges that any problem exists. It usually does not cause guilt, anxiety, or depression in the person who engages in it. Most of these people come to the attention of the nurse through an agency such as a public health department, a general hospital, or a detention home. (See Table 11, pages 230–231.)

PERSONALITY TESTS
Instruments designed to measure personality characteristics. Many are called *projective* tests because they evoke projection in the responses of the person being tested. Commonly used personality tests include the

(Text continues on page 232.)

TABLE 11. CHARACTERISTICS ASSOCIATED WITH THE MAJOR TYPES OF PERSONALITY DISORDERS

TYPE	CHARACTERISTICS
Antisocial	Behavior that causes conflicts with society such as thefts, vandalism, fighting, delinquency, truancy. Inability to sustain consistent work, to function as a responsible parent, to exhibit lawful behavior, or to maintain enduring attachment to sexual partner. Lack of respect or loyalty, irritability and aggressiveness, tendency to con others for personal gain, failure to plan ahead, tendency not to feel guilt or learn from experience and to blame others.
Avoidant	Hypersensitivity to rejection and interpretation of innocuous events as ridicule. Unwillingness to become involved with others unless given a guarantee of uncritical acceptance; social withdrawal in interpersonal and work roles: exaggerated desire for affection and acceptance, low self-esteem and overly dismayed by personal shortcomings.
Borderline	Impulsive and unpredictable in areas of life that are self-damaging, unstable but intense in interpersonal relationships, inappropriate displays of temper, mood instability, uncertainty about identity, intolerance of being alone, physically self-damaging, chronic feelings of boredom or emptiness.
Compulsive	Overconscientious, overmeticulous, perfectionistic. Excessive concern for conformity; rigid adherence to strict standards; prone to self-doubt, unhappiness, and worry; restricted ability to express warm and tender emotions; preoccupation with trivial details, rules, schedules, and lists.
Dependent	Passively allows others to assume responsibility for major areas of life. Subordinates own needs to those on whom client depends to avoid possibility of having to rely on self.

Lacks self-confidence

Histrionic	Behavior that is overly dramatic, reactive, and intense. Engages in attention seeking, self-dramatization and irrational outbursts of emotion. Perceived by others as shallow, self-indulgent, vain, demanding, dependent, inconsiderate. Prone to manipulative threats and gestures.
Narcissistic	Grandiose sense of self-importance. Preoccupied with fantasies of unlimited success, power, beauty, brilliance. Need for attention and admiration. Indifference or marked feelings of rage, inferiority, or humiliation in response to criticism. Expects special favors, takes advantage of others, shifts between overidealizing to disregard of others. Lacks ability for empathy.
Paranoid	Pervasive, unwarranted suspiciousness and mistrust evidenced by jealousy, envy, and guardedness. Hypersensitivity, usually feels mistreated and misjudged. Restricted feelings evidenced by lack of sense of humor; absence of sentimental, tender feelings; and pride in being cold and unemotional.
Passive-aggressive	Resistance to demands for adequate functioning through indirect methods such as procrastination, dawdling, stubbornness, intentional inefficiency, and forgetfulness.
Schizoid	Emotional coldness and aloofness. Indifference to praise or criticism from others. No desire for social involvement. Tendency to be reserved and seclusive.
Schizotypal	Presence of various oddities of thought, perception, speech, and behavior, such as ideas of reference, bizarre fantasies, and preoccupations. Suspiciousness and hypersensitivity to real or imagined criticism. Social isolation.

Rorschach test, the Thematic Apperception test (TAT), the Minnesota Multiphasic Personality Inventory (MMPI), the Draw-a-Person test, the Sentence Completion test, and the Bender-Gestalt test.

(*See also* Psychologic Tests)

PERVASIVE DEVELOPMENTAL DISORDER

The child suffering from a childhood onset pervasive developmental disorder is severely disturbed. This disturbance, unlike a specific developmental disorder, affects many basic areas of psychologic development. Formerly, children now classified as victims of pervasive developmental disorders may have been labeled symbiotic-psychotic or childhood schizophrenic. The onset of this full syndrome is identified later than autism, usually after 30 months and before 12 years. There are no delusions, hallucinations, incoherence, or marked loosening of associations, but the child displays an obvious and long-lasting impairment in social relationships, such as inappropriate clinging or a lack of affective response. The child also displays at least three of the following symptoms:

- Sudden excessive anxiety manifested by symptoms such as unexplained panic attacks, free-floating anxiety, or catastrophic reactions to everyday occurrences
- Constricted or inappropriate affect
- Resistance to change in environment; ritualistic behavior
- Oddities in motor movement, such as peculiar posturing
- Abnormalities of speech
- Sensitivity to sensory stimulation that is either excessive or less than normal
- Self-mutilation

Nursing Intervention

- Intensive psychotherapy and *milieu* therapy available in residential or daycare programs may be necessary.
- Therapy is usually also indicated for parents.
- Psychiatric nurses can work on a primary level of prevention by assessing and teaching parenting skills.
- Secondary level prevention includes teaching others the signs of childhood psychosis and making appropriate referrals.
- The earlier the intervention, the better the prognosis.
- Psychiatric nurses can work with severely disturbed children and their families in child guidance clinics and residential and daycare settings.

PHARMACOLOGY

(*See* Appendix **B,** Psychotropic Drugs)

PHENOTHIAZINE DERIVATIVE

A compound derived from phenothiazine that is particularly known for its antipsychotic property. Phenothiazine derivatives are among the most widely used drugs in medical practice, particularly in psychiatry.

(*See also* Appendix **B,** Antipsychotic Drugs)

PHEOCHROMOCYTOMA

A tumor of the adrenal medulla that causes excess norepinephrine production. It leads to anxiety and other personality changes that are organically determined. Physical signs—hypertension, pallor, sweating, and orthostatic hypotension—strongly suggest the diagnosis. It can be cured by surgery.

(*See also* Organic Brain Syndrome)

PHOBIA

An intense fear of some situation not ordinarily associated with danger. The phobia causes the person to
avoid the situation because of the anxiety associated
with it.

PHOBIC DISORDERS

A disorder characterized by an intense, irrational fear
of an external object, activity, or situation. It is a
response to experienced anxiety. Unlike a generalized
anxiety disorder, however, where the anxiety is free
floating, a phobia is characterized by persistent fear of
specific places or things.

Types of Phobic Disorders:

Agoraphobia. Fear of being alone or in public places.

Social phobia. Fear of situations that may be humi-
liating or embarassing.

Simple phobia. Specific fears other than the above.

Intervention Strategies

Phobic coping patterns are highly resistant to most
insight-oriented therapies since the phobic's style is
basically one of avoidance. Techniques that are commonly used include:

- *Desensitization.* Client is exposed serially to a
  predetermined list of anxiety-provoking situations
  graded in a hierarchy from least to most frightening.
  Through techniques of progressive relaxation, the
  person becomes desensitized to each stimulus in the
  scale and then moves up to the next most frightening
  stimulus. Eventually the stimulus that originally
  provoked the most anxiety no longer elicits the same
  painful response.
- *Reciprocal inhibition.* Anxiety-provoking stimulus

234

is paired with another stimulus that is associated with an opposite feeling strong enough to suppress the anxiety. Through use of tranquilizing medications, hypnosis, meditation, yoga, or biofeedback training, clients are taught how to induce in themselves both psychologic and physical calm. Once they have mastered these techniques, they are taught to use them when faced with the anxiety-provoking hierarchy of stimuli.

PHYSICAL AGGRESSION

(*See* Aggression, Physical)

PHYSICAL WITHDRAWAL

Avoidance of physical contact through missed therapy sessions, hiding, sitting far away, and so on.

Nursing Intervention

- *In severe withdrawal.* Establish contact through physical proximity; move into client's visual field (or at client's eye level); identify self; make introductory inquiry; state invitation to hear from client; state amount of time willing to stay regardless of whether client chooses to verbalize. (Encourages orientation to current external reality, the here-and-now, despite client's possible internal preoccupation)

  Give attention to client's physical needs possibly establishing initial physical bond of contact. (Enhances client's self-esteem)
- *In inpatient relationship work.* Follow through by locating client, explore absence from session in concerned manner, state availability to discuss absence; where realistic, stress necessity that client share responsibility for continuance of relationship

and change context of contract. (Interrupts dysfunctional behavioral pattern of avoidance through physical withdrawal; gives message that there are alternative behavioral patterns)

■ *In outpatient relationship work.* Follow through with outreach by phone; consider changing environmental structure in terms of time, place, or persons—for example home visits. (Interrupts dysfunctional behavioral pattern; external environmental conditions, rather than client conditions, may be an inhibiting force)

PHYSIOLOGIC AND NEUROLOGIC ASSESSMENT

The value of careful screening for physiologic disorders cannot be overemphasized in the overall assessment of the individual client. The objectives of these assessments include:

■ Detection of underlying and perhaps unsuspected organic pathology that may be responsible for psychiatric symptoms

■ Understanding of disease as a factor in overall psychiatric disability

■ Appreciation of somatic symptoms that reflect primarily psychologic rather than organic problems

History taking is an essential procedure in ruling out organic causes of psychiatric symptoms. The nurse should inquire into two primary aspects of physiologic history: (1) facts about known physical diseases and dysfunction, (2) information about specific somatic complaints.

Neurologic Assessment

A careful neurologic examination is mandatory for each client suspected of having organic brain dysfunction. Its goal is to discover signs pointing to curcumscribed, focal cerebral dysfunction or diffuse, bilateral cerebral disease. A guide for evaluating the presence of signs of central nervous system disorders is presented in Table 12 on page 236.

Explanation of Codes in Table 12

Pupils

Reaction time, right (R) and left (L)
(2) Reacts briskly
(1) Reacts slowly
(0) No reaction

Size

(=) Equal
(<) Right lesser than left
(>) Right greater than left

Level of Consciousness (L.O.C.)

(5) Alert and oriented × 3: awakens easily; oriented to person, place, time
(4) Alert and partially oriented: awakens easily but oriented in only one or two of the three spheres
(3) Lethargic but oriented: slow to arouse, possibly slurred speech, but oriented × 3
(2) Lethargic and disoriented: slow to arouse, oriented in only one or two spheres or completely disoriented

OR

(2) Restless/combative (confused): spontaneously thrashing about in bed, striking out at others, inattentive to commands
(1) Responds to stimulation only: exhibits only some type of withdrawal or posturing in response to stimulation
(0) Unresponsive: gives no response of any kind

TABLE 12. EVALUATION GUIDE FOR SIGNS OF CENTRAL NERVOUS SYSTEM DISORDERS*

TIME & DATE	PUPILS R = L ∨ ∧	L.O.C.	S-R	T.R.	MOTOR RUE	RLE	LUE	LLE	TOTAL MAX. 25'

Stimulus-Response (S-R)

(5) Responds to commands: gives appropriate responses to orientation questions, complies with instructions on hand grasp, toe wiggling, etc.

(4) Responds to name: opens eyes to name or gives some indication that he or she hears (nods, moves, etc.), but does not follow all commands

(3) Responds to shaking: responds only to vigorous physical stimulation

(2) Responds to pinprick: responds to light pain applied with pin to trunk or extremities to elicit either withdrawal or posturing

(1) Responds to deep pain: responds only to mandibular pressure, periorbital rub, sternal rub, or pinch

(0) Unresponsive: gives no response to any stimulus

Type of Response (T.R.)

(3) Complex withdrawal: withdrawal and attempt to remove stimulus

(2) Simple withdrawal: withdrawal from stimulus alone

(1) Posturing: decorticate—head, arms, and hands flexed; decerebrate—head extended, arms extended and pronated, back arched

(0) Flaccid: no response

Motor

Right Upper Extremity (RUE)
Right Lower Extremity (RLE)
Left Upper Extremity (LUE)
Left Lower Extremity (LLE)

(2) Full spontaneous use: moves designated extremity or extremities with or *without* stimulus

(1) Moves to stimulus only: responds only to touch, pin, or deep pain

(0) No movement: does not respond to any stimulus

Weakness of an extremity is indicated by writing "weaker" under the appropriate column.

*Source: Copyright © 1977. American Journal of Nursing Company. Reproduced with permission from *American Journal of Nursing,* September, Vol. 77, No. 9.

PINPOINTING

A communication skill which calls attention to certain kinds of statements, relationships, or behaviors that are similar, inconsistent, or dissimilar.

(*See also* Appendix **C,** Skills That Foster Effective Communication)

PITUITARY HYPERFUNCTION

Various types of tumors can cause increased secretion of pituitary hormones, and some of these lead to psychiatric signs and symptoms. They may be affective, behavioral, sexual (impotence, reduced libido), or perceptual/cognitive. Correct assessment is based on the presence of physical signs, especially bitemporal hemianopsia, diminished visual acuity, various endocrine organ malfunctions including hypothalamic malfunction, and perhaps the rough, enlarged facial features and hands of the classic pituitary giant. Tumors can be ablated by radiation or surgery.

(*See also* Organic Brain Syndrome)

PITUITARY HYPOFUNCTION

A tumor, an infarction, bleeding, trauma, infection, irradiation, and surgery all can lead to undersecretion of pituitary hormone. If the condition occurs from hemorrhage and shock to a postpartum mother, it is referred to as Simmonds' disease. When a client is on steroid therapy for another condition, the pituitary may be suppressed and produce too little hormone.

Clients complain of headache, appetite loss, low sexual drive, weakness, easy fatigability, irritability, and depression. They may become psychotic. Physically there is regression of sexual organs and secondary sex characteristics. The condition may be mistaken for anorexia nervosa.

(*See also* Organic Brain Syndrome)

PLAY THERAPY

The treatment modality most widely used with children, play therapy lets children use their natural medium of expression to resolve conflicts. The play therapist adds the further resource of an accepting, understanding adult. The therapist may intervene with explanations about the child's responses and behavior in language geared to the child's comprehension.

Children use play to:

- Master and assimilate past experiences that they had no control over
- Communicate with the unconscious
- Communicate with others
- Explore and experiment while learning how to relate to self, world, and others
- Compromise between the demands of drives and the dictates of reality

POST-TRAUMATIC STRESS DISORDER

Occurs when the stressor (rape or assault, military combat, kidnapping, floods, earthquakes, major car accidents, airplane crashes, bombing, torture) evokes significant distress. The syndrome appears to be more severe and to last longer when the stressor is man made.

Many people essentially "relive" the experience in

their dreams by having recurrent nightmares. Other sleep disturbances, including insomnia, often occur. Victims may feel a psychic numbing or emotional anesthesia in relationship to other people; previously enjoyed activities; and feelings of intimacy, tenderness, and sexuality. They may have difficulty in concentrating and remembering. The survivors of trauma shared with others may also feel guilty about having survived or about behavior they undertook in order to survive. When victims are exposed to situations or events that resemble or in some way symbolize the traumatic event, their symptoms may increase and they may feel even greater distress.

Three subtypes include:

1. *Acute.* Symptoms begin within 6 months of traumatic event and do not last longer than 6 months. Chances are good that person can return to a precrisis level of functioning.
2. *Chronic.* Symptoms last for 6 months or more.
3. *Delayed.* Symptoms begin after a latency period of 6 months or more.

PREMORTEM DYING
Phenomenon that may occur in interactions between a dying person and his or her family.

CHARACTERISTICS

- The dying person is less and less often allowed to participate in decisions regarding family or personal interests.
- When the terminally ill person asks questions, the family often responds: "Don't worry, everything is being taken care of."
- It generally occurs when dying is prolonged.
- While family members perceive their behavior as protecting the dying person, the behavior indicates

a change in the family system. It may imply that they no longer think of the dying person as part of the family.

- When mourning begins long before actual death, the family may finish grieving before the person dies.
- Ambivalence may be experienced by family members who begin grief work before actual death.
- Should the person recover, it may be difficult for him or her to re-enter the family system.

(*See also* Grief Work/Grieving)

PRIMARY DEGENERATION OF THE CORPUS COLLOSUM

This unusual hereditary degeneration, also known as Marchiafava's disease, occurs only in middle-aged Italian males. It seems to require a history of considerable intake of red wine. The psychiatric symptoms are dramatic manifestations of paranoia, hypomanic behavior, or, conversely, apathy progressing to dementia. Physically the motor system is impaired, there is aphasia, and convulsions occur.

(*See also* Organic Brain Syndrome)

PRIMARY DEGENERATIVE DEMENTIA

(*See* Alzheimer's Disease)

PRIMARY GAIN

Gain a person derives from the function of a symptom itself. For example, a hysterical paralysis may provide primary gain to an individual who seeks punishment for unconscious misdeeds.

PRIMARY PREVENTION

Elimination of factors that cause or contribute to the development of disease.

PRIMARY PROCESS THINKING

In psychoanalytic theory, a type of autistic mental pattern characteristic of dreams, psychosis, and early stages of life, in which logical thought processes, reality, and the restrictions of time and space are ignored.

(*See also* Psychotic Disorders)

PROBLEM-ORIENTED RECORDING

A system of recording that organizes raw data into a comprehensive whole that can be used for assessment, planning, evaluation, research, and health-care audit. It includes four elements: data base, problem list, initial plans, and progress notes. It is considered by many mental health professionals to be an improvement over the traditional source-oriented system.

PROBLEM SOLVING

A specific form of intellectual activity used when an individual faces a situation he or she is unable to handle in terms of past learning. Problem-solving strategies are considered crucial in any psychotherapeutic endeavor. They consist of the following sequential steps: observation, definition, preparation, analysis, ideation, incubation, synthesis, evaluation, and development.

PROCESSING

A complex and sophisticated communication skill in which direct attention is given to the interpersonal dynamics of the nurse-client experience. Process comments focus on the content, feelings, and behaviors experienced within nurse-client relationships.

(*See also* Appendix **C,** Skills That Foster Effective Communication)

PROJECTION

A defense or coping mechanism in which a person's own unacceptable feelings and thoughts are attributed to others.

(*See also* Defense Mechanisms)

PSYCHIATRIC AIDE

A paraprofessional who provides much of the direct service to hospitalized persons. Paraprofessionals are also being trained for and used in community mental health settings. Most receive inservice training, although community college programs for mental health workers have recently been established.

PSYCHIATRIC AUDIT

A means of appraising the quality of care received by clients of mental health services. The client's chart may be reviewed and the quality of care required compared with actual practice.

PSYCHIATRIC HISTORY

A traditional record, oriented to the medical model, designed to elicit information about an individual's previous psychiatric experiences and encounters. Information may be provided by family, friends, and others about the client, resulting in a variety of perceptions, which may differ greatly from those of the client. It is necessary to include the perceptions of the client if the data are to be meaningful from his or her viewpoint.

The psychiatric history generally includes the following information:

■ *Complaint.* The main reason the client is having a psychiatric examination (Client may have personally initiated psychiatric examination, or it may have been initiated by others.)

- *Present symptom.* Nature of onset and development of symptoms
- *Previous hospitalizations and mental health treatment.*
- *Family history.* Whether any family members have ever sought or received mental health treatment
- *Personal history.* Birth and development; past and recent illnesses; schooling and educational problems; occupation; sexual development, interest, practices; marital history; use of alcohol, drugs, tobacco; religious practices
- *Personality.* Client's relationships with others, moods, feelings, interests, leisure-time activities, and so forth

PSYCHIATRIC NURSING

A specialty within the nursing profession in which the nurse directs efforts toward promotion of mental health, prevention of mental disturbance, early identification of and intervention in emotional problems, and followup care to minimize long-term effects of mental disturbance.

(*See also* Appendix **A**)

PSYCHIATRIC SOCIAL WORKER

A graduate of a master's program in social work with an emphasis in the field of psychiatry. This professional's roles include counseling and psychotherapeutic work as well as dealing with the full range of social problems that clients and their families present.

PSYCHIATRIC TECHNICIAN

(*See* Psychiatric Aide)

PSYCHIATRIST
A physician whose specialty is mental disorders or mental diseases. Certification in psychiatry is provided by the American Board of Psychiatry and Neurology. Generally, psychiatrists are responsible for diagnosis and treatment.

PSYCHOANALYST
A physician who has undergone psychoanalytic training. Psychoanalysts are found primarily in private practice in large urban settings.

PSYCHOGENIC FUGUE
(*See* Fugue)

PSYCHOGENIC PAIN DISORDER
Pain in the absence of physiologic findings and in the presence of possible psychologic factors.

Assessment

In most clients suffering pain that may be psychologically influenced or generated, there is evidence of a stressful life situation that the client cannot handle because of particular past experiences or present states. Clues to psychogenic pain are:

- Life stress
- A complaint that is excessive for the observable injury
- Pain that is nonanatomical in distribution
- A demanding personality
- A history of repeated extensive medical-surgical procedures without relief

Intervention Involves

- Recognizing and understanding life problem or adjustment client is facing

- Recognizing and understanding client's self-perception as helpless to cope

- Helping client learn more effective ways of adapting

- Referring the client to pain clinics and support groups

PSYCHOLOGIC TESTS

Tests that are generally administered and interpreted by clinical psychologists. There are two types: intelligence tests and personality tests.

Common Psychologic Tests in Clinical Use

NAME OF TEST	DESCRIPTION	METHOD
Bender-Gestalt test	Test of visual-motor coordination that is most useful with adults as a screening device to detect presence of organic impairment. It may also be used to evaluate level of maturation in	Client is asked to copy nine separate geometric designs onto plain white paper, one at a time. Sometimes the client is asked to draw design from memory after an interval of 45–60 seconds.

NAME OF TEST	DESCRIPTION	METHOD
(Bender-Gestalt test, continued)	coordination of intellectual, muscular, and visual functions in children.	
Blacky test	Projective test used most frequently with children (although it is also designed for adults) to determine level of psychosexual development.	Client is shown various cartoons about a dog (who may be identified as male or female) and the dog's family and is asked to make up a story about each cartoon.
Draw-a-Person test	Projective test used with both adults and children to elicit information on client's body image or perception of self and relationship to environment. It is also used as a screening device to detect the presence of organic	Client is asked first to draw a human figure and later to draw a person of the opposite sex. Test may be expanded by asking client to draw a picture of a house and a tree as well (called the House-Tree-Person test), an

NAME OF TEST	DESCRIPTION	METHOD
(Draw-a-Person test, continued)	impairment. With children it may be used to compare age level of expression with child's chronologic age for a rough approximation of intelligence.	animal, or a family.
Minnesota Multiphasic Personality Inventory (MMPI)	Self-administered objective (as opposed to projective) personality test designed to yield a broad examination of personality functioning that is amenable to statistical interpretation—includes self-attitudes, certain aspects of ego functioning, and profiles of symptoms or psychopathology.	Client responds to 550 statements by indicating either "true," "false," or "cannot say." Client's personality profile is sketched in terms of: Preocupation with body diseases Depression Hysteria Antisocial personality Masculine or feminine features Paranoid qualities

NAME OF TEST	DESCRIPTION	METHOD
(MMPI, continued)		Anxiety, phobias, and psychogenic fatigue Schizophrenic features Manic features
Rorschach test	Projective test that is the most highly developed of the personality tests. It reveals personality features and symptoms and is commonly used as a diagnostic tool.	Client responds to ten cards, one at a time, consisting of black and white or colored, standardized inkblots. Responses include impressions, thoughts, and associations that come to mind while client looks at inkblot.
Sentence Completion test	Projective test designed to elicit conscious associations to specific areas of functioning to illustrate the fears, preoccupations, ambi-	Client is asked to complete spontaneously sentences such as: "I feel guilty about...," "Sex is ...," "My mother ...," "Some-

NAME OF TEST	DESCRIPTION	METHOD
(Sentence Completion test, continued)	tions, and idiosyncrasies of client.	times I wish ...," Both mood and content are noted.
Stanford-Binet Intelligence test	General intelligence test based on an age-level concept from 2 to about 15 years. It is particularly useful to test children and to evaluate mental retardation.	Client is asked to do a graded series of tasks designed to correlate with the abilities of children of a particular age group. Each set is more difficult than the one before it.
Thematic Apperception Test (TAT)	Projective test offering a standardized set of stimuli for exploring client's emotional life. Themes and interpersonal problems emerge in client's responses.	Client is shown a series of ambiguous pictures of people in various emotionally significant situations and is asked to respond by describing what is happening in the picture and telling a story about it. Adaptations have been designed for use with

NAME OF TEST	DESCRIPTION	METHOD
(TAT, continued)		children. In these, the central figure is a child or pictures of cartoon animals.
Wechsler Adult Intelligence Scale (WAIS)	General intelligence test for persons 16 years of age and older. It is the most widely used and best standardized intelligence test.	Client completes 11 subtests, which yield both verbal and performance scores as well as full-scale IQs. Subtest raw scores may also be compared to reveal variability in functioning. The subtests are: information, comprehension, arithmetic, similarities, memory for digits, vocabulary, digit symbol, picture completion, block design, picture arran-

NAME OF TEST	DESCRIPTION	METHOD
(WAIS, continued)		gement, and object assembly.
Wechsler Intelligence Scale for Children (WISC)	General intelligence test for children from 5 through 15 years of age.	Similar to the Wechsler test for adults, this test asks client to complete ten subtests, which yield separate verbal, performance, and full-scale scores.
Wechsler Memory Scale	Psychologic test for immediate, short-term, and long-term memory.	Client is asked to do seven memory tests, including current information, orientation, mental control, logical memory, digits forward and backward, visual reproduction, and associate learning. A memory quotient score is useful in the determination of organic mental syndrome.

NAME OF TEST	DESCRIPTION	METHOD
Word Association Test	Projective test similar in form and organization to the Sentence Completion test. It is designed to elicit associations to areas of conflict.	Client is asked to respond spontaneously to a series of 50 or more words, presented one at a time. Words presumed to be related to conflicts of the specific client are mixed with words that generally produce an emotional reaction.

PSYCHONEUROSIS (Neurosis)

Traditional term for a psychologic disorder in which maladaptive behavior patterns produce psychiatric distress for the individual. In DSM III, neurotic disorders are included in affective, anxiety, somatoform, dissociative, and psychosexual categories.

(*See also* Neurotic Disorders)

PSYCHOPHYSIOLOGIC DISORDER

A physical illness that is strongly influenced by psychologic problems; called a psychosomatic disorder in earlier medical-model terminology.

Stress is the common denominator in the initiation, exacerbation, or maintenance of psychophysiologic disorders. Too much stress appears to overwhelm people and increase their vulnerability to a wide range of bodily and emotional disorders. Some sources of life stress include conjugal relationships, parenting, occupational pursuits, finances, legal problems, and developmental phases.

Since stress often seems to lead to psychophysiologic disorders, reducing or overcoming stress plays an important part in their treatment. Being flexible— that is, able to change some aspect of a usual way of behaving—can often turn a potential stressor into a positive life experience.

(*See also* Rheumatoid Arthritis; Ulcer; Ulcerative Colitis)

PSYCHOSIS
A state in which a person's mental capacity to recognize reality, communicate, and relate to others is impaired, thus interfering with the person's capacity to deal with life demands.

PSYCHOSOCIAL ASSESSMENT
A dynamic process that begins in the initial contact with the client and continues throughout the nurse-client experience. Its focus is gathering social and psychodynamic data from interaction with the client to assess the client's difficulties in living rather than to formulate a psychiatric diagnosis.

(*See also* Assessment)

PSYCHOSOMATIC DISORDER
(*See* Psychophysiologic Disorder)

PSYCHOSURGERY
Surgical removal or destruction of brain tissue with the intent of altering behavior, even though there may

be no direct evidence of structural disease or damage in the brain. Marked controversy about ethical and legal questions surrounds the use of this extreme method of treatment.

The desired effect of all psychosurgery is to diminish unpleasant affects. It has little impact on disintegrative symptoms, such as hallucinations and delusions, but the client clearly is no longer threatened, frightened, or distressed by them. The same *blasé* attitude, however, carries over to the rest of the client's life, especially when large areas of the brain are removed. Clients have little feeling for members of their families, their personal appearance, socially unacceptable behaviors, and their general future. These side effects are much diminished by the newer stereotaxic methods.

PSYCHOTIC DISORDERS

A category of behavior characterized by disturbances in verbal and motor behavior that reflect problems with affect, motivation, perception, and thought.

(*See* Schizophrenia/Schozophrenic Disorder; Bipolar Affective Disorder)

Problems with Affect

PROBLEM	EXAMPLE
Change in intensity of affect. Over-response	A man responds to the death of a minor public official whom he never knew personally by weeks of mourning so intense that he is unable to work.

PROBLEM	EXAMPLE
Blunted affect	A woman recounts her recent vicious mugging with mild sadness and regret.
Lack of affect	When told that his brother has died in an accident, a man neither shows nor feels grief, shock, or relief.
Inappropriate affect. Response to an event, situation, or interaction is unsuited to stimulus	A man recalls his wife's death with good humor and laughter. A woman becomes enraged when asked if she has eaten yet.
Labile affect. Abrupt, rapid, and repeated changes in affect for no apparent reason.	Linda is watching television and laughing. She suddenly slips from the chair to the floor. Before the nurse can reach her she is up and walking down the hall cursing in a loud voice.

Nursing Intervention

- Learn to accept client's anger calmly. Client is rarely angry at nurse personally.
- Clients are influenced by social norms and so may be embarrassed by their own displays of emotion. Be alert to client's feelings about showing feelings.
- Don't encourage client to express feelings if you are not comfortable with the feelings, don't have time to listen, or are not interested.
- Don't encourage clients to express feelings unless you have a purpose in mind.

- Learn to distinguish ruminations from expression of feelings.
- Remember that emotions can be painful even to the extremely bizarre individual.
- If you are angry with these clients, tell them in a matter-of-fact way. Avoid making them feel guilty or depriving them of care.

Problems with Motivation

Client cannot, for whatever reason, recognize or control motivation (that which prompts an individual to action). Problems with motivation are recognized in regression, withdrawal, impulse behavior, hyperactivity, and ambivalence.

Nursing Intervention

- Be alert to understanding what clients tell you in whatever way they can. Take time to observe.
- Don't talk past clients or talk about them in their presence.
- Clients may not be able to stop their behavior just because you have asked them to. If behavior is not harmful to themselves or others, go away and try again later.
- Avoid using physical force by avoiding power struggles.
- Use physical force only as a last resort to protect client and others, not to make clients do what you want them to do.
- Help clients regulate their behavior to meet their needs, not yours.
- Never try to restrain even the smallest client alone.
- Remember that the client rarely wants to hurt you.

(Text continues on page 265.)

TABLE 13. PROBLEMS WITH MOTIVATION

PROBLEMS	EXAMPLE
Regression. Return to earlier and less sophisticated adaptive behavior. Regression may be to early childhood or even to infantile adaptive patterns.	Jane is a 26-year-old woman whose mother died 3 months ago. Shortly after the funeral, Jane felt frightened to be alone in her apartment and returned to her father's home. She seemed to get great comfort and satisfaction out of being in her old bedroom. She began to bring out her dolls and childhood toys. She maintained contact with her friends but spent most of her time at home caring for her father. She refused to return to work when her leave of absence was up. About a month after her mother's death, she began to carry around a favorite doll and a blanket from childhood. She was no longer doing housework but was still cooking meals for her father. She began to spend more and more time in bed with her doll and blanket. Eventually, she would not get out of bed at all. She sucked her thumb and talked to her father in a childish way. Two months after her mother's death, Jane was admitted to the hospital, mute and sucking her thumb.
Withdrawal. Retreat from life. Withdrawal may be a total break with reality. In this case the individual is no longer in touch with the real world. Withdrawal may also be an emotional (affective) break	Greg is a 23-year-old graduate student at a local university. He did well in undergraduate work and was admitted to a competitive graduate program. Shortly after his admission, he met and began living with a girl in the same program. Greg has been going to school full-time and working part-time for the last 2 years. Several months ago, he told his girl friend that he had feelings of overwhelming despair and fear and was afraid he couldn't complete the graduate program. At her insistence, he sought help at the student health

with the real world. In this case the individual is reality oriented but unable to show affective responses to external stimuli.

service. He visited with a counselor once a week for 2 months. His girl friend believed everything was going well until she came home unexpectedly and found him sitting, staring at the blank television screen. He confessed he had dropped out of school, had quit his part-time job, and was no longer talking to anyone but her and his therapist. Greg continued to stay in the apartment. He assumed the responsiblity for cleaning and cooking. He eventually quit seeing his therapist. Then he began staying up all night and sleeping most of the day. He no longer carried on conversations with his girl friend, cooked, cleaned, or watched television. He sat for hours staring into space. He finally told his girl friend that he understood the cosmic order of everything and that it was his duty to sit forever. This so frightened her that she contacted his parents. They brought him to the emergency room.

Impulsive behavior. Behavior that appears unpredictable and unmotivated by observable events. The individual is unable to exert socially expected controls and may be verbally or physically destructive, aggressive, or violent.

Billy is a 21-year-old man. He answers in monotones or not at all. He interacts only minimally. Billy spends most of his day listening to the radio with the radio very loud and very close to his ear. Suddenly he jumps up and throws the radio across the room, barely missing another client.

Joyce is a quiet 16-year-old girl. She does not interact with others. She is sitting at the dining room table eating lunch. Suddenly she gets up and starts clearing both her own and all the other clients' dishes. She is unable to stop and moves from table to table, clearing all the dishes despite attempts of clients and staff alike to prevent her. Just as suddenly she stops. She returns to her seat at the dining room table and sits staring into space.

(Continued)

TABLE 13. PROBLEMS WITH MOTIVATION (Continued)

PROBLEMS	EXAMPLE
Hyperactivity. An increase in the rate of activity. It may include emotional lability and flight of ideas.	Elizabeth is a 47-year-old, married woman. She was brought to the hospital by her husband of 25 years. Elizabeth has been hospitalized four times in the last year. She has not slept much in the last few nights. She talks incessantly and paces back and forth in the hallway. She interrupts anyone to talk about her previous hospitalizations. She cannot sit down to eat. She is labile and fluctuates from being extremely happy to being extremely sad. She can become angry at the slightest interruption in her behavior. She refuses medication because she says she feels "too good to need meds." After several attempts, the nurse gets Elizabeth to take a cup of water and her pills. Elizabeth is holding them and laughing and chatting with the nurse. In a teasing voice, Elizabeth says, "Oh, no you don't. I told you, no pills." The nurse responds, "But you need the medication." Elizabeth says angrily, "Like hell I do," and she throws the water in the cup at the nurse. Other clients laugh and so does Elizabeth. Elizabeth says, "We'll get along fine as long as you don't try to give me those pills. I really like you, dearie, I really do. Come on, and I'll help you find a towel and dry you off. I'm really sorry I did that, but you shouldn't have tried to give me the pills."
Ambivalence. Coexistence of positive and negative feelings about objects, events, situa-	Gary is a 19-year-old high school graduate brought to the hospital by his parents. His parents report that he refuses to leave his room or get a job. They seem frustrated by his behavior and are unable to deal with it any

tions, or interactions. These feelings produce the desire to do two opposite things at once. The resulting indecision is observable in exaggerated inaction, negativistic behavior, and constant action.

Exaggerated inaction. In extreme compliance (automatic obedience, robot responses), individual will not act at all unless told what to do and often how to do it.

Negativistic behavior. Individual refuses to participate. Refusal may be verbal or nonverbal or both. As ambivalent feelings intensify, individual attempts to avoid these feelings by refusing to stop, change, or start action.

longer. On the unit, Gary will do nothing unless he is told. He will stay in bed all day if he is not assisted verbally and often physically to get up. He must be told step-by-step what to do to maintain minimal functioning. He will eat only if he is told to put the bite in his mouth, to chew, and to swallow. Several weeks after admission, Gary is demonstrating less extreme compliance but has become very negativistic. He refuses to get up in the morning, and he must be physically assisted with day-to-day care. He refuses to eat but finally agrees and then refuses to stop eating. He refuses to go to occupational therapy but once there refuses to leave when the activity is over. When Gary watches television, it sometimes takes him 10 minutes to find the appropriate chair. He sits down, gets up, and sits down again. When he is finally settled, he will not move from the chair. At times, his refusal is so adamant that he sleeps in the chair through the night, and only in the morning is he able to leave it.

(Continued)

TABLE 13. PROBLEMS WITH MOTIVATION (Continued)

PROBLEM	EXAMPLE
Constant action (mannerisms, ritualistic acts, stereotyped behavior). Appears meaningless to the observer; often accompanied by repetitive speech, autism, and regression.	John is a 45-year-old man who immigrated to this country at the age of 25 after completing his degree in business administration in Mexico. He also studied flamenco dancing and still dances regularly. He was unable to find work commensurate with his education. He has been a night janitor at a large bank for the last 17 years. He has few friends and considers dancing his only interest. He was admitted to the hospital when he was found dancing in the bank lobby after his night shift. John is mute upon admission and moves his hands over his body in a continuous, ritualistic, exaggerated dance motion. The movement continues wherever he is. He is unable to eat, sleep, or use the bathroom because he cannot stop his ritualistic dance movement. John will stop if his hands and arms are restrained, but as soon as the restraints are removed, the ritualistic movements begin again.

Problems with Perception

Response of sensory receptors to external stimuli. It includes both cognitive and emotional knowledge of the perceived object, and it may include one or more of the auditory, visual, tactile, olfactory, or gustatory sensory processes. Problems may be mild and transitory, and reality orientation may be quickly regained. However, when perception is constantly disintegrating, the resulting behavior may be strange or even bizarre. The following list describes examples of problems with perception:

PROBLEMS OF PERCEPTION	SENSE	EXAMPLE
Illusions	Visual	Chairs, tables, or other inanimate objects are seen as sinister beasts.
	Auditory	The ticking of a clock is heard as a constant countdown to disaster.
	Tactile	Human flesh feels like the cold, damp skin of a toad.
	Gustatory	Water is tasted as if it were blood.
	Olfactory	Cooking meat has the smell of

PROBLEMS OF PERCEPTION	SENSE	EXAMPLE
		burning hair.
Hallucinations	Visual	Family members long dead, or God, or the Devil appear. A man sees his own death or witnesses some dreadful act being performed as if on a movie screen.
	Auditory	A woman hears the voice of God or a world-famous person (J. Edgar Hoover, Ronald Reagan) repeating her thoughts or talking about some dreadful, perverted act that she is supposed to have performed.
	Tactile	A man feels the hand of God on his shoulder. His body feels to his touch like wood or plaster.
	Olfactory	The environment is heavy with the

PROBLEMS OF PERCEPTION	SENSE	EXAMPLE
(Hallucinations, continued)		smell of death. A woman smells an offensive body odor coming from herself or others.
	Gustatory	A man tastes mother's milk in his mouth. He tastes burnt food even when he does not eat.
	Kinesthetic (somatic distortions)	The individual has strange body sensations that may or may not be part of the delusional system. A man feels as if rats or worms are crawling through his brain. A woman feels as if her heart has stopped and turned to concrete. The individual may not recognize ordinary body sensations, such as hunger or the need to urinate or defecate.

Nursing Intervention

- Don't argue about hallucinations.
- Point out your reality, but don't try to rob clients of theirs.
- Offer clients gentle reassurance.
- Don't touch clients without telling them first.
- If you are frightened by client or client's distorted perceptions, ask someone to help you.

Problems with Thought

In times of fear, stress, or anxiety, thought may not come or may not make sense. Judgment may not be reality oriented. The most common problems are in form, content, and flow of thought. The following list provides examples of problems with thought:

CHARACTERISTIC AFFECTED	PROBLEMS	EXAMPLE
Form of thought	*Symbolic associations.* Symbols such as words that should have common meanings take on specific meanings known only to individual.	Mona, a 16-year-old girl, continually runs out of cigarettes. She insists on giving them to everyone—other patients, staff, and visitors. She smokes very little herself and agrees she does not have a "real habit," but she becomes distressed, agitated, and tearful if she does not have a

CHARACTERISTIC AFFECTED	PROBLEMS	EXAMPLE
(Form of thought, continued)		pack of cigarettes stuffed in the top of her blouse. She eventually tells her primary therapist that cigarettes have always represented her heart and her love for her fellow man because she has always carried them over her heartbeat. She says that she sometimes feels drained and empty of emotion, but by giving away her cigarettes, she makes herself symbolically at one with all, and as a result, all are at one with her. She has universal love and is filled again. Cigarettes are a symbol of love and giving to Mona, not just

CHARACTERISTIC AFFECTED	PROBLEMS	EXAMPLE
(Form of thought, continued)		something to smoke.
	Concrete associations. Ability to make abstract associations and to generalize ideas is lost.	Proverb: People who live in glass houses shouldn't throw stones.
		Abstract association: You should not criticize others without expecting criticism yourself.
		Concrete association: If you throw rocks at a glass house, you will break it.
		George was continually putting all kinds of objects in the toilet and had to be accompanied to the bathroom to protect the plumbing. On one such occasion the nurse said to George, "Please let me have the book, George, and please don't put anything else in

CHARACTERISTIC AFFECTED	PROBLEMS	EXAMPLE
(Form of thought, continued)		the toilet." George entered the cubicle and urinated on the floor. He did not put *anything* else in the toilet.
	Blocking. The expression of a thought is stopped in midstream, and in a few seconds a new, unrelated thought is expressed.	Jane and the nurse are in Jane's room talking about an outing in the park. Jane says, "Parks are really lovely this time of year. The grass is all green and the flowers are starting to bloom. It's nice to take off your shoes and walk in the grass. I hope we take blankets and lots and lots ... The walls of this room are a dreadful color. Do you suppose they will ever paint them anything but this dreadful yellow? I swear I will never be able to see this color

CHARACTERISTIC AFFECTED	PROBLEMS	EXAMPLE
(Form of thought, continued)		without thinking about this room."
Content of thought	*Delusions of grandeur.* Individuals place themselves in a special relationship to the world. They may believe themselves to be prominent people, living or dead, or to be related to such people, or to be influential in important affairs.	John, a 47-year-old man raised in an orphanage with no known relatives, joined the Army during the Korean War. He received a medical discharge for psychiatric problems. At present he believes himself to be the illegitimate son of Albert Einstein. John believes that through telepathy he invented all the spacecraft for all American space fights and settled the Vietnam War. John's delusion is expansive, and he continually incorporates scientific and military advances into the system. On the whole he is a

CHARACTERISTIC AFFECTED	PROBLEMS	EXAMPLE
(Content of thought, continued)		pleasant, friendly man until his delusional system is challenged. Disagreements usually end in a fight, an arrest, and a brief hospital stay.
	Delusions of persecution. Individuals believe themselves to be harassed, in danger, under investigation, or at the mercy of some powerful force. They may be driven to drastic acts by these delusions.	Jane, a 45-year-old, unemployed schoolteacher, has always been an isolative person with few friends and few interests. When busing was begun to enforce integration, Jane believed that the school district and her fellow teachers had plotted to give her the most difficult students. Jane eventually incorporated childhood friends, relatives, and even the governor of the state into her delusional system. She resigned her

CHARACTERISTIC AFFECTED	PROBLEMS	EXAMPLE
(Content of thought, continued)		position and moved several times. Jane was hospitalized when she tried to burn down her house. Jane was discharged in 3 months with no change in her system except that she was no longer driven to act on her delusional thoughts.
	Delusions of reference. Individuals believe that certain events, situations, or interactions are directly related to themselves.	Jim, a 35-year-old man, is watching the street from the hospital window. Two people get off a city bus and walk down the street. Jim tells the nurse, "Did you see them? They are from the Symbionese Liberation Army, and now they know I'm here."
	Somatic delusions. Individ-	Lynn, a 29-year-old woman, has

CHARACTERISTIC AFFECTED	PROBLEMS	EXAMPLE
(Content of thought, continued)	uals believe that their bodies are changing or responding in some unusual way. They may be unaware of ordinary sensations such as hunger or thirst.	lost 40 pounds in the last 2 months. She had not eaten in 3 days when she was admitted to the hospital. She believes that as punishment for a secret crime, God has closed up her bowels and that if she eats she will not be able to swallow.
	Delusions of being controlled. Individuals believe that their feelings, impulses, thoughts or actions are not their own but are imposed from some external source.	David, a 20-year-old man, tells the nurse during the admission interview that he is being controlled by his father and that he can speak only when his father puts words in his mouth.
	Bizarre delusions. Content of delusion is so absurd that there is not possible way it	Mark, a 35-year-old man, is referred to psychiatry from the dentistry department, where he

CHARACTERISTIC AFFECTED	PROBLEMS	EXAMPLE
(Content of thought, continued)	could be based in fact.	reported that while he was in Vietnam a military dentist replaced the fillings in his teeth with transistors. Since then he has been the radio receiving and sending unit for all communications between the United States and China. He believes that since relations between the two countries are better, he can replace the fillings without jeopardizing the safety of the United States.
Flow of thought	*Flight of ideas.* Thoughts come so fast and bring so many associations that no single thought can be clearly expressed.	Mary approaches the nurse before dinner and says, "I hope we have chicken tonight. (Angrily) Chicken is exactly what my husband was. He called the

CHARACTERISTIC AFFECTED	PROBLEMS	EXAMPLE
(Flow of thought, continued)	Ideas occur in a rapid and endless variety of ways, connected only by a single, slim thread.	police to bring me here. (Calmly) The cops wore blue. Have you ever noticed how blue the sky is? (Happily) I'm sky-high on life and love and pursuit of happiness. Just like the constitution, not like this institution. (Angrily) This institution locks me up against the constitution. (Happily) I have rights, but right here is just fine with me."
	Retardation. Thoughts come very slowly and are difficult to express. There may be such a dearth of thought that communications are monosyllabic. There may even be mutism.	Ann explains that her thoughts are like a record being played at a slow speed.

Nursing Intervention

- If you don't understand, say so.
- Recognize the feeling, if not the content, of the communication.
- Help client regulate verbal production so you can understand.
- Listen very carefully.
- Don't argue or agree with delusions.
- Remember that really understanding disintegrative communications takes a long time and lots of patience.

PSYCHOTROPIC DRUGS

(*See* Appendix **B**)

QUESTIONING

A very direct communication activity that may be useful when the nurse needs specific information from the client.

(See also Appendix **C,** Skills That Foster Effective Communication)

R

RAPE
Forced sexual intercourse without the partner's consent. The legal definition of rape as a crime varies from state to state. A distinction is made between statutory rape, involving the seduction of a minor, and forcible rape, in which the victim is over 18 years of age.

Rape Prevention Counseling generally emphasizes three strategies:

1. Women should avoid isolated areas. Women who are alone should avoid being helpful to strangers.
2. A woman who is attacked should resist from the beginning unless her life is being threatened. Screaming, running away, or fighting back may induce a would-be rapist to look for a more cooperative and easily intimidated victim.
3. If the assailant has a knife or gun, however, the woman who resists risks being injured or killed. In such cases it is sometimes wiser to submit.

   The physical consequences of rape include injury, pregnancy, and venereal disease. The emotional consequences include the trauma associated not only with the experience itself but also with the humiliation of the legal procedures. Nursing interventions can offer rape victims information and psychological support.

RATIONALIZATION
A defense or coping mechanism in which a person falsifies experience by constructing logical or socially approved explanations of behaviors.

(See also Defense Mechanisms)

REACTION FORMATION

A defense or coping mechanism in which unacceptable feelings are disguised by repression of the real feeling and reinforcement of the opposite feelings.

(See also Defense Mechanisms)

REACTIVE ATTACHMENT DISORDER OF INFANCY

The primary symptom or characteristic of this disorder (sometimes referred to as "failure to thrive") is a lack of emotional and physical development or growth in the infant over a period of time. A physiologic etiology, such as heart, central nervous system, or kidney abnormality, must be ruled out. Therefore, hospitalization and evaluation of physiologic functioning are essential. If no physiologic etiology can be isolated, the problem may be due to psychologically inadequate caretaking. During hospitalization, a nurturing plan is developed for the infant, using specifically assigned personnel and involving the caretaker parent. If the infant grows and develops with nurturing, it is usually concluded that a reactive attachment disorder of infancy exists, with problems of parenting as a causative factor. Frequently, psychotherapeutic and child protective interventions are necessary.

REALITY TESTING

The ability to differentiate one's thoughts and feelings from the outside world. Psychological introspection is considered a sophisticated form of reality testing. Impaired reality testing results in opinions that are based not on validated exerience but on emotional needs that block accurate perception of reality.

(See also Psychotic Disorders)

RECIPROCAL INHIBITION

The technique of pairing an anxiety-provoking stimulus with another stimulus that is associated with a feeling of opposite quality strong enough to suppress the anxiety.

(*See also* Behavior Modification)

REFLECTING

A communication skill in which the nurse reiterates either the content or the feeling message of the client. In *content* reflection, the nurse repeats basically the same statement as the client. In *feeling* reflection, the nurse verbalizes what seems to be implied about feelings in the client's comments.

(*See also* Appendix C, Skills That Foster Effective Communication)

REGRESSION

A coping mechanism whereby the individual reverts to earlier patterns of behavior.

(*See also* Defense Mechanisms)

REPRESSION

A coping mechanism in which unacceptable feelings are kept out of awareness.

(*See also* Defense Mechanisms)

REQUESTING ILLUSTRATION

A communication skill in which the client is asked to give an example to clarify a meaning in order to help the nurse understand better.

(*See also* Appendix C, Skills That Foster Effective Communication)

RESISTANCE

All the phenomena that interfere with and disrupt the smooth flow of feelings, memories, and thoughts. In the traditional psychoanalytic sense, anything that inhibits the patient from producing material from the unconscious.

Resistance inevitably surfaces in the course of one-to-one work as client begins to address self-defeating, nonintegrated aspects of self. It is often mistakenly seen as the client's struggle against the nurse. It actually is the client struggling against change, against modifying behavior patterns. Although these old behavior patterns may have self-defeating aspects, they have also provided some satisfaction or protected against discomfort. Thus, a client may resist giving up a defense that offered protection from the anxiety associated with unbearable thoughts and impulses.

The nurse must exercise caution in evaluating a client's behavior as resistive. Resistance to specific topics or concerns may mean that the client is not yet ready for investigative work.

Assessment

Behaviors that may be suspected as resistance include:

- Forgetting events
- Focusing on the past to avoid talking about the present (or vice versa)
- Consistent avoidance of certain topics or inquiries
- Antagonism toward, or falling in love with, therapist
- Acting out
- Acting in

Nursing Intervention

- First, be aware of resistance.

- Label resistive behavior with client.
- Allow resistance to occur several times to demonstrate its presence to client.
- Explore accompanying emotion and history of its development.
- Facilitate working through the resistance by fully understanding and appreciating its implications in client's life.

(*See also* Defense Mechanisms)

RETARDATION OF THOUGHT
A condition in which thoughts come very slowly and are difficult to express. There may be such a dearth of thought that communications are monosyllabic. Mutism may be observed in severe retardation of thought.

(*See also* Mental Status Examination; Psychotic Disorders)

REVERSAL
A coping mechanism in which the person manifests an instinctual wish by the opposite action, thought, or feeling (also called inversion).

RHEUMATOID ARTHRITIS
Long identified as an illness that is strongly influenced by emotional life, it is a progressive inflammatory disease primarily of the joints, with unknown causes.
  Associated personality traits include:

Overcontrolled

Highly responsible

Sensitive to criticism

Self-sacrificing

Criteria for identification include physical findings,

such as deformities and subcutaneous nodules, and blood studies.

(*See also* Psychophysiologic Disorders)

RIGHTS OF CLIENTS

(*See* Legal Aspects)

RITUALISTIC ACTS

Constant action behavior that appears meaningless to the observer, often accompanied by repetitive speech, autism, and regression.

(*See also* Compulsion)

RORSCHACH TEST

A personality test in which a person says whatever comes to mind as he or she looks at a series of ten standardized cards with inkblots on them (also called inkblot test). It is believed to reveal many aspects of the individual's personality structure and emotional functioning.

(*See also* Psychologic Tests)

S

SCAPEGOATING

Process in which one member of a family or group is blamed for misfortunes and problems. The scapegoat is given the role of whipping post, draining off the family or group system's feelings of guilt and inadequacy.

Assessment

Scapegoating is common in many groups, particularly adolescent groups. It occurs in three stages:

1. Frustration generates aggression.
2. Aggression becomes displaced upon relatively defenseless others.
3. Through blaming, projecting, and stereotyping, this displaced aggression is rationalized and finally justified.

Nursing Intervention

- Refrain from attempting merely to rescue scapegoat (target of hostile remarks) since this may augment the anger and frustration of other clients.
- Ask group (or family) to focus on what is going on, to acknowledge the anxiety or other uncomfortable feeling that preceded the scapegoating.
- Anticipate scapegoating in times of stress and attempt to circumvent process before it gets out of control.
- Be aware that scapegoats share some responsibility for their predicament by presenting themselves to others in a different or provocative stance.

SCHIZOID

Characterized by withdrawal, daydreaming, and detachment. The individual appears shy, seclusive, solitary, and sensitive. Such a person is usually viewed by others as eccentric. The essential feature of a schizoid personality is a defect in the capacity to form warm, tender relationships.

(*See also* Personality Disorders)

SCHIZOPHRENIA/SCHIZOPHRENIC DISORDER

Diagnostic term for a disintegrative life pattern characterized by thinking disorder, withdrawal from reality, regressive behavior, poor communication, and impaired interpersonal relationships. Four symptoms ("the four As") are considered classic: (a) disturbances in association, (b) flattened affect, (c) ambivalence, and (d) autism. The term is criticized by some mental health professionals as a label that tends to elicit the disturbed functioning from an individual over time.

DIAGNOSTIC CRITERIA FOR SCHIZOPHRENIC DISORDER*

1. At least one of the following during a phase of the illness:
   a. Bizarre delusions (content is patently absurd and has no possible basis in fact), such as delusions of being controlled, thought broadcasting, thought insertion, or thought withdrawal
   b. Somatic, grandiose, religious, nihilistic, or other delusions without persecutory or jealousy content
   c. Delusions with persecutory or jealousy content if accompanied by hallucinations of any type
   d. Auditory hallucinations in which either a voice keeps up a running commentary on individual's

*Source: The American Psychiatric Association, Diagnostic and Statistical Manual of Mental Disorders, Third Edition, Washington, D.C., A.P.A. 1980. Reprinted by permission.

behavior or thoughts, or two or more voices converse with each other

e. Auditory hallucinations on several occasions with content of more than one or two words, having no apparent relation to depression or elation

f. Incoherence, marked loosening of associations, markedly illogical thinking, or marked poverty of speech content if associated with at least one of the following:

Blunted, flat, or inappropriate affect

Delusions or hallucinations

Catatonic or other grossly disorganized behavior

2. Deterioration from a previous level of functioning in such areas as work, social relations, and self-care

3. Duration: Continuous signs of illness for a least 6 months at some time during the person's life, with some signs of illness at present. The 6-month period must include an active phase during which there were symptoms from 1 above, with or without a prodomal or residual phase, as defined below.

Prodromal phase. A clear deterioration in functioning before the active phase of the illness due neither to a disturbance in mood nor to a substance use disorder and involving at least two of the symptoms noted below.

Residual phase. Persistence, following the active phase of the illness, of at least two of the symptoms noted below, due neither to a disturbance in mood nor to a substance use disorder.

Prodomal or Residual Symptoms:

a. Social isolation or withdrawal

b. Marked impairment in role functioning as wage earner, student, or homemaker

c. Markedly peculiar behavior (collecting garbage, talking to self in public, or hoarding food)

d. Marked impairment in personal hygiene and grooming

e. Blunted, flat, or inappropriate affect

f. Digressive, vague, overelaborate, circumstantial, or metaphorical speech

g. Odd or bizarre ideation, or magical thinking such as superstitiousness, clairvoyance, telepathy, "sixth sense," "others can feel my feelings," overvalued ideas, ideas of reference

h. Unusual perceptual experiences, such as recurrent illusions, sensing presence of a force or person not actually present

4. Full depressive or manic syndrome, if present, developed after any psychotic symptoms, or was brief in duration relative to duration of psychotic symptoms in 1 above.

5. Onset of prodromal or active phase of illness before age 45.

6. Not due to organic mental disorder or mental retardation

(*See also* Psychotic Disorders)

SCHIZOPHRENIFORM

May look like, but is not, true schizophrenia. It meets all criteria for schizophrenia except duration: Illness (including prodromal, active, and residual phases) lasts more than 2 weeks but less than 6 months. It is neither long-term nor persistently disintegrative; the person will probably recover fully and have no residual impairment. In true schizophrenia, the course is long-term and persistently disintegrative.

SCHIZOTYPAL PERSONALITY DISORDER

Characterized by social isolation, but clients experience social anxiety or hypersensitivity to real or imagined criticism; suspiciousness; magical thinking;

ideas of reference; recurrent illusions; and vague, circumstantial and metaphorical speech patterns.

(*See also* Personality Disorders)

SCHOOL PHOBIA

Actually not a phobia but an acute anxiety reaction related to separation from home and major attachment figures. Child displays a sudden and seemingly inexplicable fear of going to school and/or complains of many physical symptoms on school days. If child is allowed to stay home, the dread of returning to school usually increases. Child and parent should have psychiatric intervention quickly (before the problem becomes worse) to help child separate from parent. Separation anxiety disorder can manifest itself by: reluctance or refusal to go to school, reluctance to go to sleep, avoidance of being alone in the house, unrealistic worries about the safety of major attachment figures and/or that untoward events will separate the child from the major attachment figure, nightmares about separation, sadness or apathy when not with the major attachment figure, and signs of excessive distress (for children under 6, this must be of panic proportions to qualify as a symptom of separation anxiety disorder) when anticipating separation from major attachment figures. The duration of the disturbance must be at least 2 weeks for the child to be diagnosed as suffering from a separation anxiety disorder.

SECONDARY GAIN

The social and psychological uses a client may make of symptoms, for example, gaining sympathy, psychological support, financial advantages, or special treatment by virture of being labeled ill.

SECONDARY PREVENTION
The early detection and treatment of disease.

SELECTIVE INATTENTION
A filtering out of stimuli under conditions of moderate and severe anxiety.

(*See also* Anxiety)

SELF-ACTUALIZING
Defined by Abraham Maslow as making full use of one's talents and potentials; doing the best one is capable of doing.

SELF-AWARENESS
A sense of knowing what one is experiencing. It is a major goal of all therapy, individual and group.

SELF-CONCEPT
A person's image of self, usually the conscious image.

SELF-DEPRECATION, DELUSIONS OF
(*See* Delusions)

SELF-ESTEEM
One's feeling of value, worthiness, or competency.

SELF-FULFILLING PROPHECY
A phenomenon in which an individual, through selective inattention, distorts his or her perceptions of another and then gradually develops mannerisms and behavioral traits that cause the other to relate to him or her as expected. The interpersonal distortion thus becomes self-perpetuating.

SENTENCE COMPLETION TEST

(*See* Psychologic Tests)

SEPARATION ANXIETY

An infant or child's fear and apprehension upon being removed from the parent figure. A parallel process occurs in the termination phase of a nurse-client therapeutic relationship, as the client relives the anxiety associated with childhood loss of the supportive figure.

There are three phases in the separation anxiety experienced by hospitalized children:

1. *Protest.* This first stage lasts from a few hours to several days. Children in this stage still consciously need mother and expect that their efforts to regain her will succeed. They still hope that mother will meet their needs as she has in the past. Need for mother and terror at losing her produce an anxiety that sharply reduces the child's perceptual field. Behavioral manifestations of this stage include loud crying, screaming, tossing around in bed or crib, focusing eagerly on any sight or sound that might be the mother, and rejecting the attentions of others.

2. *Despair.* In this stage the child still consciously needs mother but no longer expects that efforts to regain her will succeed. Crying is now intermittent or monotonous, replacing the screams of rage and terror characteristic of the protest stage. The despairing child is apathetic and listless and does not interact with the environment.

3. *Detachment.* In this stage, children use the defense mechanism of repression to deal with their intense anxiety. They repress their need of the mother, often to the point of not seeming to recognize her when she

visits. At this stage the child does not cry when mother leaves and does interact with the environment. The child in anaclitic depression is in the final stages of the detachment phase.

Children who have reached the detachment phase are often erroneously believed to have adjusted to the hospital situation. Actually, these children have lost faith in their parents' love and ability and willingness to protect them. This loss of faith has obvious implications for their readjustment on returning home. It may also affect how they will handle terminations and separations for the rest of their lives.

SEXUALITY/SEXUAL ASSESSMENT/SEX THERAPY

Stages of Sexual Response

PHASE	RESPONSE
Excitement	Muscle tension increases (myotonia), particularly in striated muscles of arms and legs. May be some tensing in smooth muscles of abdomen late in phase. Heart rate and blood pressure increase moderately. Sex flush (more common in females) may appear late in phase. Nipple erection occurs (with greater reliability in females).
Plateau	Myotonia becomes quite pronounced throughout the body. Heart reate increases just before orgasm; blood pressure continues to ele-

PHASE	RESPONSE
(Plateau, continued)	vate. Breathing becomes faster and deeper. Sex flush becomes more pronounced or may appear at this phase.
Orgasm	Involuntary muscle spasm occurs throughout body with reduction in voluntary muscle control. Blood pressure and heart rate reach highest levels. Hyperventilation and heart rate peak. Sex flush, if present, usually persists through orgasm. External rectal sphincter muscle contracts involuntarily.
Resolution	All signs of myotonia are absent usually within 5 minutes after orgasm. Heart rate, blood pressure, and breathing rate begin to return to normal. Nipple erection subsides slowly (more rapidly in females).

Sexual problems associated with illnesses can be classified into four general groups:

1. Disinterest in or lack of desire for sexual activity
2. Physical incapacity for or discomfort during sexual activity
3. Fear of precipitating or aggravating a physical illness through sexual activity
4. Use of illness as an excuse to avoid feared or undesired sexual activity

Sexual Problems and Medical-Surgical Conditions

MEDICAL-SURGICAL PROCEDURE/CONDITION	ASSOCIATED SEXUAL DIFFICULTIES
Sterilization without hormonal therapy	Loss of potency and low sperm counts
Prostatectomy	Retrograde ejaculation and loss of urethral phase of orgasm
Perineal prostatectomy	Impotency and loss of urinary control
Ostomies	Disorders of potency
Bilateral oophorectomy	Loss of libido

Sexual Problems Related to Various Conditions

CONDITION	COMMONLY OCCURRING SEX-RELATED PROBLEM
Mental retardation	Limitation to sexual behaviors such as individual and mutual masturbation
	Risk of being sexually exploited by others
Organic brain syndromes	Occasional bizarre hypersexuality
	Loss of social control with retreat toward more primitive sex behaviors at inappropriate times or circumstances
	Decreased interest in

CONDITION	COMMONLY OCCURRING SEX-RELATED PROBLEM
(Organic brain syndromes, continued)	sexual activity due to related depression
Affective disorders	Decreased libido and potency associated with depression
	Increased incidence of promiscuity during manic episodes
	Increased sexual preoccupation during manic episodes
	Sexual delusions
Psychotic disorders	Sex often associated with unusual patterns and variations
Nonpsychotic clinical syndromes	Sexual inhibitions
Personality disorders	Sexual indifference with hysterical life styles
	Sexual offenses associated with compulsions; promiscuity
Aging	Menopausal women may experience lack of vaginal lubrication, less frequent and less intense orgasm, and less sexual desire
	Men may not wish to ejaculate as often, may experience difficulty

CONDITION	COMMONLY OCCURRING SEX-RELATED PROBLEM
(Aging, continued)	maintaining erections, and may find that their erections are less firm
Taking medications	Antihypertensives, psychotropics, antidepressants, antispasmodics, sedatives, tranquilizers, and narcotics may all impair clients' ability to perform sexually
Use of alcohol	Alcoholism is associated with impotence and the man's ability to achieve an erection. Women may experience a decline in ability to experience an orgasm or to become aroused.
General stress from job or living situation	Sexual performance anxiety that includes sweating, nausea, palpitations, and hyperventilation
Lack of affection	May result in sexual disinterest

Assessment

A suggested format for a sexual assessment interview*:

1. Open the discussion of sexual matters subtly with

an open-ended question. "People with your illness or stresses often experience other difficulties, sometimes with sexual functioning."

2. Follow-up with another open-ended question about client's current status. "Has your illness or stresses made any difference in what it's like for you to be a wife or husband (lover, boyfriend, girlfriend, sexual partner)?"

3. If the client speaks of having a dysfunction, ask about its effect. "How does this affect you?" or "How do you feel about it?"

4. Ask about the severity and duration of the dysfunction. "Is it always difficult to control your ejaculation?" "Tell me when you first noticed this."

5. Ask about the effects on client's sexual partner. "Has this affected your relationship with your partner?"

6. Ask what client has already done to alleviate the situation. "Have you made any adjustments in your sexual activity?"

7. Ask client if and how he or she would like the situation changed. "How would you like to change the situation to make it more satisfying?"

*Source: Adapted from M.P. Whitley and D. Willingham, "Adding a Sexual Assessment to the Health Interview," *Journal of Psychiatric Nursing and Mental Health Services,* Vol. 16, No. 4, April 1978, pp. 17-27.

Interventions for Sexual Difficulties*

SEXUAL DIFFICULTY	GUIDELINES FOR THERAPEUTIC INTERVENTION
Premature ejaculation Man tends to ejaculate before woman has an orgasm.	A climate of comfort and acceptance for sexual interaction is re-established
	Client is encouraged to

SEXUAL DIFFICULTY	GUIDELINES FOR THERAPEUTIC INTERVENTION

(Premature ejaculation, continued)

masturbate and enjoy touch and body stimulation in general.

Man or woman is instructed to stimulate the erect penis until premonitory sensations of impending orgasm are felt. Then penile stimulation is abruptly stopped. This process is repeated to train threshhold of excitability to be more tolerant of stimuli. Sometimes woman uses "squeeze technique," in which at the point of orgasm she squeezes the head of the penis with thumb and first two fingers for 3–4 seconds. This stops the urge to ejaculate.

Couple is also instructed in ways to reduce tactile component of friction in the vagina by limiting frequency of thrusts or extent of movement within the vagina.

Primary impotence
Man has never been able to maintain an erection sufficient to accomplish sexual intercourse.

Intercourse is avoided, and nongenital caressing exercises begin with man and woman alternating as initiators of a session of caressing,

SEXUAL DIFFICULTY

(Primary impotence, continued)

Secondary impotence
Man currently cannot maintain or even get an erection but has had a history of past successful entries. The occasional impotence that most men experience because of tiredness or distraction is not considered secondary impotence.

Primary orgasmic dysfunction
Woman has never had an orgasm by any method.

Situational orgasmic dysfunction
Woman is able to have orgasms under certain conditions and at certain times but not others. For example, she may be able to masturbate to orgasm but not achieve orgasm during intercourse.

GUIDELINES FOR THERAPEUTIC INTERVENTION

thus sharing responsibility for sexual interaction.

Next, genital stimulation is added to provide the couple with positive sexual experiences without intercourse.

When intercourse is attempted, woman is instructed to assume superior position and insert man's penis into her vagina.

When setbacks occur, couple is advised to rely on sexual techniques that do not involve intercourse.

Couple is advised to assume a nondemanding position for female stimulation.

Woman is to place her hand lightly on her partner's to indicate her preference for contact.

Emphasis is not on achieving orgasm but on learning erotic preferences.

Couple is instructed to use the lateral side-by-

SEXUAL DIFFICULTY	GUIDELINES FOR THERAPEUTIC INTERVENTION

(Situational orgasmic dysfunction, continued)

side position, which enables both partners to move freely with emphasis on slow, exploratory thrusting.

Goal is to develop an ability to enjoy pelvic play with penis inside vagina.

Functional vaginismus Involuntary tightening or spasm occurs in outer third of vagina that can be so severe as to make intercourse impossible.

Initial step is physical demonstration of her involuntary vaginal spasm to woman by inserting an examining finger into her vagina.

Then Hegar dilators in graduated sizes are inserted by man into woman's vagina. At first she manually controls his insertion of smallest dilator. Later he can insert larger dilators following her verbal instructions.

After larger dilators are successfully inserted, she is instructed to retain dilator for several hours each night. Most involuntary spasms can be relieved in 3 to 5 days with daily use of dilators.

In addition to physical

SEXUAL DIFFICULTY	GUIDELINES FOR THERAPEUTIC INTERVENTION
(Functional vaginismus, continued)	relief from spastic constriction, therapy is directed toward alleviating the fear that led to onset of symptoms.

*Source: Compiled from Masters, W., and Johnson, V., 1970. *Human Sexual Inadequacy* Boston: Little, Brown and Co., pp. 30-56.

SHALLOW AFFECT

Indicated by an insufficiently intense emotional display in associaton with ideas or situations that ordinarily would call for a more adequate response; also called flattening of affect.

(See also Mental Status Examination)

SHAPING

An intervention designed to change a client's behavior.

(See also Behavior Modification)

SILENCE

(See Verbal Withdrawal)

SITUATIONAL DISORDERS

Diagnostic classification for transient mental health disturbances that are not psychotic in nature. These disturbed reactions are considered to result from overwhelming environmental stress although what is overwhelming may differ greatly from one individual to another.

(See also Traumatic Stress Disorder)

SLEEPWALKING DISORDER

A person with this disorder exhibits an altered state of conscious awareness of the surroundings resembling sleep. Such people often have valid recollections of emotionally traumatic events that they have consciously forgotten.

(*See also* Dissociative Disorder)

SOCIOTHERAPY

A treatment mode emphasizing environmental, social, and interpersonal factors rather than intrapsychic factors.

SODIUM AMYTAL INTERVIEWS

(*See* Narcotherapy)

SOMATIC DELUSIONS

(*See* Delusions)

SOMATIZATION DISORDER

Clients with this disorder have sought medical attention for recurrent and multiple somatic complaints of several years duration, but there is no evidence of physical disorder. This problem usually begins before the age of 30 and has a chronic course often accompanied by anxiety and depressed mood. Clients believe they have been sickly for a good part of their lives and report lengthy lists of symptoms including blindness, paralysis, convulsions, nausea, and painful menstruation.

(*See also* Somatoform Disorder)

SOMATOFORM DISORDER

Characterized by physical symptoms suggesting physical disorders for which there is no positive evidence.

Nursing Intervention

Once organic problems and factitious disorders have been ruled out and a client's behavior is confirmed as representing an example of a somatoform disorder, the following guidelines may be used to plan an intervention strategy:

- Be aware of personal responses to client. Many nurses find people who employ physical symptoms irritating to deal with. Often these people are self-centered, self-indulgent, and manipulative. Nurses who cannot cope with their own reactions to these clients cannot work with them effectively. It may help to remember that these clients do not intentionally produce their symptoms, nor do they appreciate the effect their behavior has on other people.

- Try to avoid reinforcing client's symptoms. "Ignore the symptoms but never the client." To concentrate on physical symptoms is giving the symptoms more attention than they merit, thus increasing secondary gain.

- Assess the symbolic meaning of client's symptoms. People who cope with anxiety by converting it into hysterical physical symptoms have difficulty communicating verbally. The nonverbal communication function of the symptom should be considered. The common symptoms of blindness, deafness, pain, numbness, itching, swelling, vomiting, paralysis, and so forth may be communicating somethng as general as: "Take care of me," "Pay attention to me," or "I want out of these responsibilities."

SOMATOTHERAPY
The treatment of emotionally disturbed or incapacitated clients by physiologic means.

(*See also* Biologic Therapies)

SOMNAMBULISM

(*See* Dissociative Disorders; Sleepwalking Disorders)

STANFORD-BINET SCALE
A commonly used intelligence test for children consisting of a series of tasks of increasing difficulty.

(*See also* Psychologic Tests)

STRUCTURING
A communication skill directed toward creating order or evolving guidelines. A nurse may structure content or structure the parameters of the nurse-client relationship.

(*See also* Appendix **C,** Skills That Foster Effective Communication)

SUBACUTE COMBINED DEGENERATION
Combined systems disease affects both motor and sensory systems of the central nervous system. Its cause is insufficient absorption of vitamin B_{12}, as in the disease pernicious anemia. The mental changes run the gamut of organically induced psychiatric syndromes, from irritability and negativism to paranoia, memory loss, and frank psychosis. Clients also complain of numbness and tingling in the extremities and pain in the legs. They exhibit loss of position and vibration sense, positive Romberg sign, spastic-ataxic gait, either hyperreflexia or hyporeflexia, and prematurely

grey hair. Genetic factors contribute to incidence, as the disease occurs more commonly in blue-eyed Scandinavian females than in any other group, and runs in families. Treatment is with vitamin B_{12}.

(*See also* Organic Brain Syndrome)

SUBDURAL HEMATOMA

A person who is suffering from bleeding around the surface of the brain may present a confusing clinical picture, and misdiagnosis may prove fatal. Especially when the onset is rather insidious, accurate recognition may be difficult. Bleeding may occur in an elderly person after a small injury to the head, and all that may be detectable is irritability, occasional memory lapses, and periodic mutism. The condition can progress, however, to loss of consciousness, coma, and death. Physical signs of a subdural hematoma include papilledema, unequal pupils, hemiparesis on the opposite side, increased deep tendon reflexes, and positive Babinski's reflex. Electroencephalograms, roentgenograms, brain scans, computerized axial tomography (CAT) scans, and possibly arteriography may be needed to establish and localize the lesion.

(*See also* Organic Brain Syndrome)

SUBLIMATION

A coping mechanism in which unacceptable drives are diverted into personally and socially acceptable channels.

(*See also* Defense Mechanisms)

SUBSTANCE USE DISORDERS

Conditions in which a person:

1. Requires a certain drug to maintain his or her functioning.

2. Develops a tolerance for it requiring increased doses.
3. Develops physical withdrawal symptoms if the drug is stopped.
4. Psychologically feels that it is impossible to get along without drug.

Assessment

The following personality traits are often associated with disruptive drug use:

- Dominant and critical behavior with underlying self-doubts and passivity
- Tendency to describe own parents as self-reliant and efficient but not emotionally warm
- Personal insecurity
- Problems with sexual identification
- Rebellious attitudes toward authority
- Tendency to use defense mechanisms that are primarily escapist
- Inability to form close and lasting affection ties
- Absence of strong and efficient superego
- Marked narcissistic trends

To assess a client who is abusing drugs, it is important to collect the following data:

What drug is being used?

How much is being used on a daily basis?

How frequently is it used?

How long has client been using it?

What combination of drugs is being used?

Nursing Intervention

STEP	KEY CONSIDERATIONS
1. Assessment of drug use pattern.	Find out what drug or drugs are being used.

STEP

(Assessment, continued)

KEY CONSIDERATIONS

For each drug, note

Quantity on a daily basis

Frequency of use

Duration of use

Collect data to establish whether alcohol is being used in combination with other sedative-hypnotics.

Remember that more accurate information may be obtained by interviewing client's parents or friends, or by a physical exam and blood and urine lab tests, than by questioning client directly.

2. Support during detoxification or withdrawal

Gradual withdrawal or detoxification is essential for persons addicted to barbiturates, nonbarbiturate hypnotics, and tranquilizers. Abrupt withdrawal can be fatal.

Detoxification takes from 2–3 weeks and should take place in a structured inpatient setting.

Phenothiazines may be

STEP	KEY CONSIDERATONS

(Support, continued)

used as an adjunct to treatment.

Nurse should attend to accompanying physical problems, such as abcesses at injection sites, hepatitis, malnutrition, and respiratory and gastrointestinal disease.

It may be necessary to give verbal reassurance and reality orientation to reduce feelings of panic during withdrawal. It is essential to stay with person who is on a bad trip until effects of drug wear off.

Fatigue and depression lasting for several weeks accompany withdrawal from stimulants.

3. Rehabilitation

Long-range treatment is based on helping person learn better mechanisms for coping with stress and problems.

In programs such as methadone treatment, nurse may need to learn to administer methadone and supervise such med-

STEP	KEY CONSIDERATIONS
(Rehabilitation, continued)	ical procedures as collecting and processing of urine samples.
	Selection of clients for a long-term rehabilitation program should be based on a thorough evaluation of individual. Not all drug users are hardcore junkies. Rehabilitation programs exist for drug experimenters and social users as well as for established addicts.

(*See also* Alcohol/Alcoholic/Alcoholism)

SUBSTITUTION

A coping mechanism in which a person replaces an unacceptable wish, desire, emotion, or goal with one that is more acceptable.

(*See also* Defense Mechanisms)

SUICIDE

The taking of one's own life. It is considered destructive aggression turned inward. Suicide has evoked many myths. Some examples are:

MYTH	REALITY
A suicide threat is just a bid for attention and should not be taken seriously.	All suicidal behavior should be taken seriously; a bid for attention may be a cry for help.

MYTH	REALITY
It is harmful for a person to talk about suicidal thoughts. The person's attention should be diverted when this occurs.	Of prime importance in planning nursing care is an accurate assessment of the lethality of the person's suicide plan.
Only psychotic persons commit suicide.	The majority of successful suicides are committed by persons who are not psychotic.
People who talk about suicide won't do it.	Most people do talk about their suicide intention before making a suicide attempt.
A nice home, good job, or an intact family prevents suicide.	Complex sociocultural, physiologic, or psychologic stressors may all be related to suicide.
A failed suicide attempt should be treated as manipulative behavior.	Failed suicide attempts are more likely to be evidence of a person's ambivalence toward killing himself or herself.

Variables Regarding Suicide Rates

VARIABLES	HIGHER RATES	LOWER RATES
Social	Societies in which social unrest, internal governmental problems, or pessimistic outlooks for the	Developing communities and groups in which hope and optimism are high

VARIABLES	HIGHER RATES	LOWER RATES
(Social, continued)	future predominate	
	Cultures that are uncaring and cold and lack concern for people in trouble, such as skidrows and disorganized inner-city areas	Cultures that are warm and nurturing, such as Irish, Italian, and Norwegian
	Societies, such as the United States, Japan, Russia, and Germany, that value independence and individual performance	Areas in which there is strong disapproval of suicide as an act, such as Italy, Spain, and Ireland, where the Catholic Church is highly influential
	Social roles, occupations, and professions in which people exhibit high concern and nurturance toward others (physicians and police, for example)	

VARIABLES	HIGHER RATES	LOWER RATES
Demographic	Single people and married people without children	
	Men in general, although rates have increased 49% for white women and 80% for black women in the the past 20 years	
	White people, although the rate for young, urban black persons between 20 and 35 years of age is twice that of white persons in the same age group	
	Persons above the age of 40, although rates for adolescents are rising (persons over 65 account for 25% of the total number of reported suicides)	

VARIABLES	HIGHER RATES	LOWER RATES
Clinical	People who have attempted suicide before	
	People who have experienced the loss of both parents early in life, or the loss of or threat of loss of their spouse, job, money, or social position	
	People who are depressed or recovering from depression or a disintegrative life pattern	
	People with physical illness, particularly when the illness involves an alteration of body image or lifestyle	
	People who abuse alcohol and drugs, thus decreasing their impulse control	

Assessment

- People bent on suicide almost always give either verbal or nonverbal clues of their intent.
- When the message is indirect or subtle ("I just can't take it anymore," "Take care of my cat and dog"), just as when the message is direct, it is a cry for help.
- Sometimes behavior provides the clue: giving away prized possessions, making a will, or cancelling social engagements are examples.
- Once clues have been identified, the next step is to undertake an accurate lethality assessment.

Nursing Intervention

- These clients must be protected from themselves. This may involve phoning a poison control center, taking steps for immediate intervention by a crisis team, enlisting client's family to help, or removing dangerous objects on an inpatient unit.
- Inpatient clients should be carefully observed once the environment has been made safe.
- The mental health team makes the determination of when immediate suicidal danger is over.
- Suicidal risk increases for depressed clients once they begin to feel somewhat better and more energetic.
- Long-term goal is to provide suicidal client with continued supports both through therapeutic relationships and through a network of family, relatives, friends, or community groups.

(See also Lethality Assessment)

SUMMARIZING

A communication skill in which main ideas are highlighted. Summarizing reviews for client and nurse what the main themes of the conversation have been. It is useful in helping the client to focus thinking.

(*See also* Appendix **C**, Skills that Foster Effective Communication)

SUPPRESSION
A defense or coping mechanism in which unacceptable feelings and thoughts are consciously kept out of awareness.

(*See also* Defense Mechanisms)

SYDENHAM'S CHOREA
Patients who have rheumatic fever as children may develop Sydenham's chorea in their teens. It occurs more often in females. The mental symptoms, which can be dramatic in severe cases, may be the initial complaints. These range from apathy and irritability to what appears to be a manic episode. The physical signs are rapid shaking of the tongue, palate, and extremities, protrusion of the tongue, and facial grimacing. Onset of the syndrome may be provoked by pregnancy, and the condition may be mistaken for a bizarre conversion hysteria secondary to pregnancy during adolescence.

(*See also* Organic Brain Syndrome)

T

TARDIVE DYSKINESIA

A disorder characterized by involuntary movements of the face, jaw, and tongue, resulting in bizarre grimacing, lip smacking, and protrusion of the tongue. The syndrome frequently occurs after years of antipsychotic drug treatment. It is generally irreversible, although it can be modified through adjustment of medication.

(*See also* Appendix **B**, Antiparkinsonian Agents)

TERTIARY PREVENTION

The elimination or reduction of residual disability following illness.

THEMATIC APPERCEPTION TEST

(*See Psychologic Tests*)

THOUGHT DISORDER

A condition in which associations tend to lose their continuity so that thinking becomes confused, bizarre, incorrect, and abrupt.

(*See also* Mental Status Examination; Psychotic Disorders)

TRANQUILIZING DRUGS

A drug that depresses central nervous system function in a highly selective manner, exerting a calming effect without appreciably impairing the person's level of awareness. Major tranquilizer is synonymous with antipsychotic drug.

(*See also* Appendix **B**, Antipsychotic Drugs)

TRANSACTIONAL ANALYSIS (TA)

A system introduced by Eric Berne that has four components: (1) structural analysis of intrapsychic phenomena, (2) transactional analysis proper, (3) game analysis, and (4) script analysis. TA is used in both individual and group psychotherapy.

TRANSCENDENTAL MEDITATION (TM)

A learned meditation technique originally developed by the Maharishi Mahesh Yogi. In TM a person may sit with eyes closed for two 20-minute sessions every day, concentrating on a mantra (a word or sound believed to possess mystical power). The object is to relieve tension and to improve bodily feeling and interpersonal relationships.

TRANSFERENCE

In psychoanalytic theory, an unconscious phenomenon in which feelings, attitudes, and wishes originally linked with significant figures in one's early life are projected onto others who have come to represent these figures in one's current life. Transference may be viewed as a distortion in interpersonal contact based on unresolved conflicts from client's past relationships.

Nursing Intervention

- Accept client's reactions. (Maintains contact in the best therapeutic interests of the client)
- Encourage client to develop awareness of source of transference. (May free client to deal with nurse as individual separate from original transference figure)
- Consider termination of relationship work if negative transference appears unresolvable and client

risks further dysfunction. (Termination preferable to escalating dysfunction)

TRICYCLICS

The most commonly used class of antidepressant drugs. Tricyclics are close in chemical structure to the phenothiazines and have many similar side effects, but they have profoundly different effects on mood, behavior, and cognition. They are not antipsychotic when given to schizophrenic patients and may aggravate a psychosis.

(*See also* Appendix **B**, Antidepressant Drugs)

TUBEROUS SCLEROSIS

Epiloia or tuberous sclerosis is a disease of the myelin sheaths of nervous tissue in which lesions are scattered throughout the brain. Distinctive physical signs include skin lesions consisting of swollen sebaceous glands that appear over the nose and cheeks as bumps. In addition to intellectual retardation and seizures, clients may exhibit psychotic symptoms. Adolescents are frequently affected, and there appears to be a familial tendency.

(*See also* Organic Brain Syndrome)

U

ULCER

Peptic ulcer, especially duodenal ulcer, has been one of the most thoroughly studied psychophysiologic illnesses. Ulcer is the classic example of a disorder in which physical and psychologic factors interact by means of feedback loops—that is, physical processes (in this instance, gastric hypersecretion) contribute to psychologic processes that influence or determine the stressful circumstances under which the client suffers pathophysiologic changes. Frustration and stress in later life increase gastric secretion which in turn leads to an incresed risk of peptic ulcer formation.

(*See also* Psychophysiologic Disorders)

ULCERATIVE COLITIS

A classic example of a lower bowel disorder with psychophysiologic characteristics. In this disease of the large intestine, a psychologically traumatic event can precipitate severe inflammatory changes in the mucosa of the intestinal wall leading to ulceration and bleeding. This disorder tends to be chronic, with remissions and relapses. It seldom disappears, exhibiting the same lasting characteristics as the personality constellation associated with it.

ASSOCIATED PERSONALITY CHARACTERISTICS

Neatness

Orderliness

Punctuality

Indecisiveness

Emotional guardedness

Humorlessness

Conscientiousness

Obstinateness

Conformity

Overintellectuality

Moral rigidity

Worry

(*See also* Psychophysiologic Disorders)

VALUES CLARIFICATION

A systematic method of teaching the process of valuing. Its strategies and exercises engage the learner in becoming aware of personal beliefs and values, choosing among alternatives, and matching stated beliefs with actions.

VERBAL THREATS

Threatened aggressive contact.

Nursing Intervention

- Continue, rather than avoid, client contact. (Interrupts dysfunctional behavior pattern)
- Explore threat or frustration that preceded indication of hostility. (Focuses on thinking, rather than action, and encourages identification of feelings)
- Allow time and space for client to verbalize feelings (helplessness, inadequacy, anger) associated with threat or frustration. (New experience may be laden with anxiety)
- Encourage client to make connections between specific threat or frustration, subsequent feelings, and specific manifestation of hostility. (Allows analysis of client's mode of conflict resolution)
- Explore client's possible need for external controls such as medication or exercise; assess degree of closeness tolerated by client. (Sets limits regarding threatened aggressive contact)
- Provide consistent set of expectations about and guidance toward self-control. (Respects personal choice, yet emphasizes expectation for self-control)

(See also Aggression)

VERBAL WITHDRAWAL

Avoidance of contact through silence or, in its extreme form, mutism.

Nursing Intervention

- Explore "what is said" by silence. (Silence may have numerous meanings—resistance, pause before emotive content, and so forth)
- Maintain attitude of continued interest. (Avoids rejection or punitive maneuvers that client may typically experience from others because of silence)
- Show acceptance of client's silent self-expression. (Silence is nonverbal communication: "I don't choose to talk now")
- Alter communication techniques: Use painting, music, or letter writing. (Opens up communication through alternate channels)
- Consider a no-demand approach in cases of mutism. (Empathic approach to say "I'm with you:" underlines client's freedom to speak or remain mute)

VIOLENCE

(See Aggression)

VOLUNTARY COMMITMENT

The legal process by which a person chooses to be admitted to a mental hospital. It requires written application by the person or by someone acting in his or her behalf, such as a parent or guardian.

(See also Legal Aspects)

W

WECHSLER ADULT INTELLIGENCE SCALE

(See Psychologic Tests)

WECHSLER INTELLIGENCE SCALE FOR CHILDREN

(See Psychologic Tests)

WECHSLER MEMORY SCALE

(See Psychologic Tests)

WERNICKE-KORSAKOFF SYNDROME

Syndrome resulting when the thiamine deficiency of excessive alcohol use leads to lesions in the midbrain (also called Wernicke's encephalopathy). Classically, on physical examination there is paralysis of lateral gaze of the external ocular muscles, nystagmus, ptosis of the eyelids, tremor, ataxia, dysmetria, and visual problems. On mental status examination, the client may appear apathetic, indifferent, and disoriented; suffering memory loss, hallucinations, or confusion. Thiamine is therapeutic.

(See also Korsakoff's Syndrome; Organic Brain Syndrome)

WIFE BATTERING

(See Family Violence)

WILSON'S DISEASE

Hepatolenticular degeneration, or Wilson's disease, is caused by deficient metabolism of copper, which then accumulates in the central nervous system, eyes, and brain. This is generally a familial disease. Dysfunction of the basal ganglia of the brain gives rise to extrapyramidal tract symptoms, such as muscular rigidity, flapping tremor of the arms, and masklike face. A greenish-brown ring around the cornea of the eye, the Kayser-Fleischer ring, confirms the diagnosis. Cirrhosis of the liver occurs. Behavior abnormalities may be dramatic, closely resembling schizophrenia. Chelating drugs, which bind copper and promote excretion, may alleviate some of the damage.

(*See also* Organic Brain Syndrome)

WITHDRAWAL

A behavior pattern characterized by avoidance of contact. It may be functional or dysfunctional in nature. Withdrawal may be avoidance of interpersonal relationships and/or a sense of reality.

(*See also* Physical Withdrawal; Verbal Withdrawal)

WORD ASSOCIATION TEST

(*See* Psychologic Tests)

APPENDIX A

1982 ANA STANDARDS OF PSYCHIATRIC AND MENTAL HEALTH NURSING PRACTICE

PROFESSIONAL PRACTICE STANDARDS

Standard 1   Theory

The nurse applies appropriate theory that is scientifically sound as a basis for decisions regarding nursing practice.

Standard 2   Data Collection

The nurse continuously collects data that are comprehensive, accurate, and systematic.

Standard 3   Diagnosis

The nurse utilizes nursing diagnoses and/or standard classification of mental disorders to express conclusions supported by recorded assessment data and current scientific premises.

Standard 4   Planning

The nurse develops a nursing care plan with specific goals and interventions delineating nursing actions unique to each client's needs.

Standard 5   Intervention

The nurse intervenes as guided by the nursing care plan to implement nursing actions that promote, maintain, or restore physical and mental health, prevent illness, and effect rehabilitation.

Standard 5A   Psychotherapeutic Interventions

The nurse uses psychotherapeutic interventions to assist clients in regaining or improving their previous coping abilities and to prevent further disability.

Standard 5B   Health Teaching

The nurse assists clients, families, and groups to achieve satisfying and productive patterns of living through health teaching.

Standard 5C   Activities of Daily Living

The nurse uses the activities of daily living in a goal-directed way to foster adequate self-care and physical and mental well-being of clients.

Standard 5D   Somatic Therapies

The nurse uses knowledge of somatic therapies and applies related clinical skills in working with clients.

Standard 5E   Therapeutic Environment

The nurse provides, structures, and maintains a therapeutic environment in collaboration with the client and other health care providers.

Standard 5F   Psychotherapy

The nurse utilizes advanced clinical expertise in individual, group, and family psychotherapy, child psychotherapy, and other treatment modalities to function as a psychotherapist, and recognizes professional accountability for nursing practice.

Standard 6   Evaluation

The nurse evaluates client responses to nursing action in order to revise the data base, nursing diagnoses, and nursing care plan.

PROFESSIONAL PERFORMANCE STANDARDS

Standard 7   Peer Review

The nurse participates in peer review and other means of evaluation to assure quality of nursing care provided for clients.

Standard 8   Continuing Education

The nurse assumes responsibility for continuing education and professional development and contributes to the professional growth of others.

Standard 9   Interdisciplinary Collaboration

The nurse collaborates with other health care providers in assessing, planning, implementing, and evaluating programs and other mental health activities.

Standard 10   Utilization of Community Health Systems

The nurse participates with other members of the community in assessing, planning, implementing, and evaluating mental health services and community systems that include the promotion of the broad continuum of primary, secondary, and tertiary prevention of mental illness.

Standard 11   Research

The nurse contributes to nursing and the mental health field through innovations in theory and practice and participation in research.

APPENDIX B

PSYCHOTROPIC MEDICATIONS

COMMONLY USED PSYCHOTROPIC DRUGS

TRADE NAME	GENERIC NAME	DRUG CATEGORY
Akineton	Biperiden	Antiparkinsonian drug
Artane	Trihexyphenidyl	Antiparkinsonian drug
Atarax	Hydroxyzine	Antianxiety agent
Aventyl	Nortriptyline	Tricyclic antidepressant
Benadryl	Diphenhydramine	Antiparkinsonian drug Antianxiety agent
Cogentin	Benztropine	Antiparkinsonian drug
Dalmane	Flurazepam	Hypnotic agent
Doriden	Glutethimide	Hypnotic agent
Elavil	Amitriptyline	Tricyclic antidepressant
Equanil	Meprobamate	Antianxiety agent
Haldol	Haloperidol	Antipsychotic agent
Kemadrin	Procyclidine	Antiparkinsonian drug

TRADE NAME	GENERIC NAME	DRUG CATEGORY
Librium	Chlordiazepox-ide	Antianxiety agent
Lithium	Lithium Carbonate	Antimania drug
Loxitane	Loxipine	Antipsychotic drug
Marplan	Isocarboxazid	Monoamine-oxidase (MAO) inhibitor
Mellaril	Thioridazine	Antipsychotic drug
Miltown	Meprobamate	Antianxiety agent
Moban	Molindone	Antipsychotic drug
Nardil	Phenelzine	MAO inhibitor
Navane	Thiothixene	Antipsychotic drug
Nembutal	Phenobarbital	Hypnotic agent
Noctec	Chloral hydrate	Hypnotic agent
Noludar	Methyprylon	Hypnotic agent
Norpramin	Desipramine	Tricyclic anti-depressant
Parnate	Tranylcypro-mine	MAO inhibitor
Pertofrane	Desipramine	Tricyclic anti-depressant
Placidyl	Ethchlorvynol	Hypnotic agent
Prolixin	Fluphenazine	Antipsychotic drug
Quaalude	Methaqualone	Hypnotic agent

TRADE NAME	GENERIC NAME	DRUG CATEGORY
Ritalin	Methylpheni-date	Central nervous system stimulant
Seconal	Secobarbital	Hypnotic agent
Sinequan	Doxepin	Tricyclic anti-depressant
Stelazine	Trifluoperazine	Antipsychotic drug
Taractan	Chlorprothix-ene	Antipsychotic drug
Thorazine	Chlorpromaz-ine	Antipsychotic drug
Trofranil	Imipramine	Tricyclic anti-depressant
Trilafon	Perphenazine	Antipsychotic drug
Valium	Diazepam	Antianxiety agent
Vistrail	Hydroxyzine	Antianxiety agent
Vivactyl	Protriptyline	Tricyclic anti-depressant

PRINCIPLES OF ADMINISTERING PSYCHOTROPIC DRUGS TO THE AGED

NURSING RESPONSIBILITIES

■ Guide decisions regarding drugs with accurate observation of need. Inexact impressions are dangerous.

- Educate clients and observe for potentially hazardous side effects.
- Use minimum amounts of medication and increase dosage only when necessary.
- Give sufficient time to assessing response to a drug rather than prematurely switching to another.
- Confer with physicians regarding specific reason for selecting and prescribing a certain drug.
- Alert physicians to total drug profile of an individual, including over-the-counter drugs that are habitually used and alcohol intake. Hazardous interactions are frequent.
- Encourage periodic lab tests to monitor cumulative toxicity.
- Encourage physicians to discontinue all but life-sustaining medications for the first week of hospital stay. Medications may be the source of symptoms.
- Use interpersonal contact and comfort measures before resorting to use of hypnotics or minor tranquilizers.
- Accurately record drugs given and reactions.

NURSING CONCERNS

- Tranquilizers in conjunction with diuretics increase incidence of hypotension, confusion, and incontinence.
- Hypnotics increase incidence of incontinence, confusion, and falls.
- Tricyclics may cause urinary retention and cardiac complications.
- Minor tranquilizers increase problems of mobility in persons with an unsteady gait.
- Cumulative reactions, including tardive

dyskinesia, are more frequent among the aged taking major tranquilizers.

- Depression, confusion, and paradoxic agitation may be due to psychoactive drugs.
- Reduced smooth muscle mobility and mucoid secretions that occur in normal aging are increased by the use of major tranquilizers.
- Tranquilizers (major and minor) and hypnotics may lower body temperature to dangerous levels in the aged who are prone to hypothermia.
- Many psychoactive drugs increase intraocular pressure and reduce visual accommodation. This is dangerous for persons with glaucoma and those with already poor visual accommodation.
- The aged are more vulnerable to lithium and tricyclic toxicity because of impaired renal filtration and clearance.

ANTIANXIETY DRUGS

Effects The antianxiety agents—sedatives and hypnotics—have very similar pharmacologic attributes. All, in fact, can be used in small or modest doses to relieve anxiety and in larger doses to induce sleep. Although they share the major clinical effect of tranquilization or disinhibition of fear-induced behavior, their side effects, including their addictive potentials and overdose sequelae, make certain representatives of this class more suitable for routine use and others better to reserve for limited, special circumstances.

The antianxiety agents are sometimes referred to as "minor tranquilizers," but this is a misleading term, since their effects on anxiety are qualitatively, not quantitatively, different from those of the "major tranquilizers" or antipsychotic agents.

There is considerable evidence that Generalized Anxiety Disorder (which is manifested by steady, continuous, and persistent anxiety symptoms) responds well to the benzodiazepine drugs.

Prior to treatment with antianxiety agents, however, medical conditions that may present symptoms of anxiety must be ruled out. A thorough history and physical exam are thus necessary prerequisites to antianxiety drug therapy. Among the medical conditions associated with anxiety symptoms are angina pectoris, allergic reactions, drug intoxications or withdrawal, caffeinism, temporal lobe epilepsy, hyperventilation, hypoglycemia, asthma, mitral valve prolapse, paroxysmal atrial tachycardia, pulmonary embolus, hyperthyroidism, pheochromocytoma, pain, hemorrhage, and electrolyte imbalance.

Benzodiazepines

The major class of drugs today in the management of anxiety is the benzodiazepines. This group, represented by chlordiazepoxide (Librium) and diazepam (Valium), accounts for a very high percentage of all the psychoactive medications prescribed in the United States by psychiatrists and medical practitioners alike. The major side effects of the benzodiazepines are related to their sedative qualities.

Use in Reducing Anxiety   There is no question that Librium and Valium offer a rather rapid, effective, and safe treatment for the emotional state commonly known as anxiety. In contrast to all other sedatives with proved effectiveness, the benzodiazepines have a low physiologic addiction potential, have never been solely responsible for a fatality from overdose, and do not interfere with or accelerate the metabolism of medications taken concurrently.

TABLE 14. DOSAGE RANGE OF ANTIANXIETY DRUGS

CLASS	GENERIC NAME	TRADE NAME	USUAL DOSAGE RANGE
Benzodiaze-pines	Chlordiaze-poxide	Librium	5-25 mg tid* or qid†
	Diazepam	Valium	2-10 mg bid‡ or qid
Propane-diols	Meproba-mate	Miltown Equanil	400mg tid or qid
Antihista-mines	Diphenhy-dramine	Benadryl	25-50 mg tid or qid
	Hydroxy-zine	Vistaril Atarax	25-50 mg tid or qid

*Three times daily
†Four times daily
†Twice daily

Drug Information Card for Antianxiety Agents (Health Teaching)*

ANTIANXIETY AGENTS (VALIUM, LIBRIUM, TRANXENE, SERAX, OXAZEPAM, VISTARIL)

Action: Decreases anxiety

Side Effects/Precautions:

1. You may experience drowsiness or dizziness while taking this medication.
2. Avoid the use of alcohol or other depressant drugs while taking this medication. The use of alcohol or other drugs should be discussed with your doctor.
3. You may be lightheaded or dizzy when standing up from a lying or sitting position. If this occurs, sit

*From drug cards written by Janet E. Smith RN, MSN

down until the dizziness passes and then stand up slowly.

4. Do not drive a car until you are sure the medication does not make you drowsy.

5. Do not abruptly stop taking this medication unless directed by your doctor.

Your drug is ——————————————————————

Your dosage is ——————————————————————

ANTIDEPRESSANT AGENTS

Antidepressant drugs are generally indicated for specific types of depression. People diagnosed with melancholia appear to have the most predictable response to these drugs. They suffer from the following symptoms:

- Severely depressed mood
- Loss of interest
- Inability to respond to normally pleasurable events or situations
- Depression that is worse in the morning and may get slightly better as the day goes on
- Early morning awakening (and the inability to fall asleep again)
- Marked psychomotor retardation or agitation
- Significant anorexia and weight loss
- Excessive or inappropriate guilt

In some other cases of depressed mood, antidepressant drugs are not effective. Thus, accurate diagnosis is necessary to ensure maximum effectiveness.

Delayed Reaction A significant, and commonly overlooked, clinical consideration is that antidepressants have a *delayed reaction onset*. Thus, a client will not show lessening of depressed mood until a week to 10

TABLE 15. ANTIDEPRESSANT DRUGS*

CLASS	GENERIC NAME	TRADE NAME	STARTING DOSE (mg/DAY)	EFFECTIVE DOSE RANGE (mg/DAY)	MAINTENANCE (mg/DAY)
Tricyclics					
Dibenzazepines	Imipramine	Tofranil	75	150–300	150
	Amitriptyline	Elavil	75	150–300	150
	Desipramine	Norpramin, Pertofran	75	150–250	150
Dibenzocycloheptenes	Nortriptyline	Aventyl	40–75	40–100	100
	Protriptyline	Vivactyl	15	15–60	30
Dibenzoxepins	Doxepin	Sinequan	75	75–300	150
Monoamine-oxidase inhibitors	Tranylcypromine	Parnate	20	20–60	20
	Isocarboxazid	Marplan	10	20–60	20
	Phenelzine	Nardil	15	45–90	45
Central nervous system stimulants	Dextroamphetamine	—	5	5–30	—
	Methamphetamine	—	2.5	2.5–20	—
	Methylphenidate	Ritalin	10	10–60	—

*Source: Compiled in part from Hollister, L. E. 1973. *Clinical Use of Psychotherapeutic Drugs.* Springfield, Ill.: Charles C Thomas, Publisher, p. 97.

338

days following the institution of an adequate dose of tricyclics.

Special Syndromes Treated with Antidepressants

- Spontaneous panic attacks often leading to agoraphobia have been shown to respond much more effectively to imipramine (Tofranil) than to the usual drug treatments of anxiety.
- Syndromes characterized by high levels of anxiety associated with depression, have often been treated with the tricyclic doxepin (Sinequan), which combines antidepressant and antianxiety effects. Triavil, a combination of perphenazine (Trilafon) and amitriptylene (Elavil) has also been used.
- The stimulant drugs amphetamine and methylphenidate have been used with success in the treatment of hyperactivity in children suffering from attention deficit disorders.

Tricyclics

The most commonly used class of antidepressant drugs is the tricyclics. These compounds are close in chemical structure to the phenothiazines and have many similar side effects but profoundly different effects on mood, behavior, and cognition.

Use in Schizophrenia Tricyclic antidepressants are not antipsychotic agents when given to schizophrenic persons and may, in fact, aggravate a disintegrative pattern or precipitate overt symptoms in a client with latent disintegrative behavior. The phenothiazines, on the other hand, do exert some antidepressant activity.

Tricyclic Side Effects Many of the common side effects of tricyclic drugs are autonomic, due to their anticholinergic characteristics. These would include dry mouth, blurred vision, constipation, palpitations, and urinary retention. Clients with glaucoma must be treated with caution. Some allergic skin reactions have been observed. Tricyclics also cause changes in the normal electrical conduction of the heart, which is particularly significant in treating persons with a history of cardiovascular disease, especially heart block. Sudden death has occurred during tricyclic treatment. Clients with known heart disease and most elderly clients thus require electrocardiograms before initiation of tricyclic therapy and periodically during the course of treatment. Several other central nervous system effects may occur including tremor, twitching, paresthesias, ataxia, and convulsions.

Drug Information Card for Tricyclic Antidepressants (Health Teaching)*

TRICYCLIC ANTIDEPRESSANTS (Elavil, Tofranil, Norpramine, Triavil (perphenazine plus amitriptyline), Sinequan)

Action: Antidepressant

Side Effects/Precautions:

1. You may experience a dry mouth, blurred vision, constipation, or drowsiness while taking this medication.
2. It may take up to 3 or 4 weeks before you begin to feel less depressed, but it is essential that you continue to take this medication as directed by your doctor, even though you do not feel any positive effect.
3. Avoid the use of alcohol and other depressant drugs while taking this medication, unless directed by your physician.
4. Do not drive a car until you are sure the medication does not make you drowsy.

*From drug cards written by Janet E. Smith RN, MSN.

5. You may be lightheaded or dizzy when standing up. Standing up slowly will help to prevent this. In the morning when you awaken, sit up in bed for one full minute before standing.

6. Notify your doctor if you become constipated or have difficulty passing urine. Use of a stool softener such as dioctyl sodium sulfosuccinate (Colace), may be beneficial if you are constipated.

Your drug is ⎯⎯⎯⎯⎯⎯⎯⎯⎯⎯⎯⎯⎯⎯⎯⎯

Your dosage is ⎯⎯⎯⎯⎯⎯⎯⎯⎯⎯⎯⎯⎯⎯⎯

Overdose Effects   The consequences of an overdose during tricyclic treatment are rather serious. Significant overdoses may cause delirium, hyperthermia, convulsions, and even coma, shock, and respiratory failure. Drug intake deserves close attention since many of the clients treated with these drugs are severely suicidal. Serious overdosage is a medical emergency and may require heroic resuscitative measures. When the nurse reports delirium and peripheral autonomic symptoms of anticholinergic poisoning due to mild overdosage, the psychiatrist can intervene with intravenous or intramuscular physostigmine (0.2 or 0.4 mg), an anticholinesterase that will reverse the delirium and other symptoms at least transiently.

MAO Inhibitors

Some clients who do not respond to tricyclic antidepressants may respond to the other major class, the monoamine-oxidase (MAO) inhibitors. These drugs generally are not as effective as tricyclics and are somewhat slower to act, sometimes requiring a month or two of treatment before improvement shows. Iproniazid (Marsilid) is considered the most effective, with

(Text continues on page 346.)

TABLE 16. COMMON SIDE EFFECTS OF ANTIDEPRESSANT MEDICATIONS*

SIDE EFFECT	INTERVENTION	SIDE EFFECT	INTERVENTION
Anticholinergic		*Psychiatric*	
Dry mouth	Encourage frequent sips of water. Suggest lemon juice and glycerine mouth swabs, dietetic or nonsucrose sourball candies, or a commercial oral lubricant.	Anxiety, restlessness, irritability	Advise physician, as dose may need to be decreased or increased or time of administration changed; medication may need to be changed to one that produces more sedation, such as amitriptyline; sedatives and/or antipsychotics may be required.
Constipation	Encourage intake of bran, fresh fruits and vegetables, and prunes. Maintain adequate fluid intake. Suggest stool softeners or laxatives. Withhold medication and advise physician, as urecholine may be needed to prevent para-	Hypomania	Withhold medication and inform physician, as antidepressant may be unmasking a bipolar disorder.
		Mental confusion, psychotic behavior	Discontinue drug; physostigmine (antidote for

Side Effect	Nursing Intervention
	...lytic ileus when constipation is severe.
Urinary retention and delayed micturition	Monitor intake and output. Check for abdominal distention. Withhold medication and advise physician if client unable to void; catheterization and/or urecholine may be required.
Blurred vision	Assure client that this is temporary. Suggest eye consult if persists beyond medication adjustment period (about 3 weeks).
Diaphoresis	Encourage adequate fluid intake (preferably noncaloric) to replace lost fluid. Observe for symptoms of electrolyte imbalance.

Neurologic

Side Effect	Nursing Intervention
	severe anticholinergic side effects).
Drowsiness	Advise client initially not to operate hazardous machinery. Administer medication at bedtime. If persistent, advise physician, as medication may need to be changed to a less sedative antidepressant.
Lowering of seizure threshold	Observe seizure precautions during initial treatment. Advise physician if seizure occurs, as adjustment of anticonvulsant in clients with seizure disorders and/or

(Continued)

TABLE 16. COMMON SIDE EFFECTS OF ANTIDEPRESSANT MEDICATIONS (Continued)

SIDE EFFECT	INTERVENTION	SIDE EFFECT	INTERVENTION
(Anticholinergic, continued)		*(Neurologic, continued)*	discontinuation of antidepressant may be warranted.
Atropine psychosis	Withhold medication and advise physician, as medication must be discontinued.	Fine tremor and/or ataxia	If severe, stop medication and advise physician, as change in dose or medication may be needed.
Cardiovascular Tachycardia	Monitor pulse for rate and arrhythmias. Withhold medication and notify physician if resting pulse rate is faster than 120.	*Endocrinologic/ Metabolic* Decreased or increased libido	Assure client that this is usually transitory. If persistent or interfering with compliance, advise physician, as change in medication and/or dose may be indicated.
Orthostatic hypotension	Record blood pressure with client sitting and standing; withhold medication and notify physician if systolic blood pressure drops more than 20-30 Hg.		

Arrhythmias and T-wave abnormalities	Monitor pulse for irregularities. Provide for routine electrocardiogram (ECG) and serial ECGS if client has history of conduction defects.
Ejaculatory and erection disturbances	Advise physician if this interferes with compliance, as medication or dose may need changing.
Weight gain	Monitor weight. Counsel client to eat nutritionally balanced adequate diet.

*Adapted from "Antidepressant Drug Therapy," by M. D. DeGennaro et al., copyright, 1981, American Journal of Nursing Company. Reproduced, with permission, from American Journal of Nursing. Vol. 81, No. 7 (July 1981).

phenelzine (Nardil) and tranylcypromine (Parnate) slightly behind. (Iproniazid is not available in the United States, however.)

What complicates the decision to use MAO inhibitors is that they are associated with several very severe side effects. Hepatic necrosis, commonly fatal, and hypertensive crises leading to intracranial bleeding are among the most threatening. This latter reaction, heralded by symptoms of severe headache, stiff neck, nausea, vomiting, and sharply increased blood pressure, follows the ingestion of foods that contain the amino acid tyramine and of sympathomimetic medications.

Clients taking tricyclics and MAO inhibitors conjointly have also occasionally had severe reactions, with fever, convulsions, and even death. Therefore, a 7- to 10-day washout period is recommended between these types of medications. Under experienced guidance and control, however, they can be prescribed simultaneously.

Substances Causing Hypertensive Crises with MAO Inhibitor Treatment*

FOODS TO AVOID		DRUGS TO AVOID
Cheddar or other aged cheese	Coffee	Amphetamine
	Licorice	Dextroamphetamine
	Pickles	
Beer	Sauerkraut	Methylamphetamine
Wine (particularly Chianti)	Smoked salmon (lox)	
		Ephedrine
Chicken liver	Snails	Dopamine
Yeast products	Raisins	Phenylpropanolamine
Broad beans	Figs	
Pickled herring	Soy sauce	Caffeine

FOODS TO AVOID	DRUGS TO AVOID
Chocolate	Epinephrine
Yogurt	

*Source: Compiled in part from Appleton, W. S. and Davis, J. M. 1973. *Practical Clinical Psychopharmacology* New York: Medcom Press, pp. 114–115.

Drug Information Card (Health Teaching) MAO Inhibitors*

MAO INHIBITORS (Parnate, Nardil)

Action: Antidepressant

Side Effects/Precautions:

1. It is essential that you continue to take this medication as directed by your doctor, even though you do not feel any positive effect. It may take up to 3 or 4 weeks before you begin to feel less depressed.
2. You may be lightheaded or dizzy when standing up. Standing up slowly will help to prevent this. In the morning when you awaken, sit up in bed for one full minute before standing.
3. Do not use alcohol while taking this medication.
4. Some foods contain a substance (tyramine) that may cause a serious increase in your blood pressure while taking this medication. Do not eat the following:

Beer	All types of liver
Canned figs	Meat tenderizer
Chianti wine	Pickled herring
Cheese	Pods of broad beans
Chocolate	(fava beans)

*From drug cards written by Janet E. Smith RN, MSN.

Raisins	Sour cream
Bananas or avocados	Soy sauce
Sherry	Yeast extracts

5. Do not use large amounts of caffeine in any form (coffee, tea, cola).
6. Many medications used in combinations with MAO inhibitors can increase your blood pressure. These include other types of antidepressants, cough and cold preparations, and sedatives. Do not take any over-the-counter products without consulting your doctor or pharmacist. Tell any doctor you visit that you are taking an MAO inhibitor.
7. Notify your doctor if you become constipated or have difficulty passing urine. Use of a stool softener such as dioctyl sodium sulfosuccinate (Colace) may be beneficial if you are constipated.
8. Report any of the following symptoms to your doctor: headache, stiff neck, nausea, or dizziness.
9. Your doctor or pharmacist may give you an ID card which states that you are taking an MAO inhibitor. Carry this with you at all times.

Your drug is _____

Your dosage is _____

The principles for use of both tricyclic and MAO inhibitor antidepressants are:

- Drug treatment does not preclude psychotherapy, electroconvulsive therapy, or behavioral treatments if they are also indicated.
- Tricyclic treatment should be given first unless there are contraindications, clinical indications for MAO inhibitors, or a past history of tricyclic antidepressant unresponsiveness.
- The usual therapeutic range is 150–300 mg per day.

Dosages may be variable and may be limited by significant side effects.

■ A response is seen 2 or 3 weeks after the therapeutic dose is reached.

■ Clients with recurrent major depressive episodes with melancholia may require long-term maintenance treatment, although doses are usually lower than those needed in acute episodes.

Other Drugs

Stimulants, such as amphetamines and methylphenidate (Ritalin), and the phenothiazines are less commonly used antidepressants. Stimulants are not a proven treatment. Phenothiazines may be particularly useful in the presence of agitation. Some clinicians and researchers believe that major depressive episodes with psychotic features (delusional depressions) respond better to a combination of an antidepressant and an antipsychotic agent or to electroconvulsive therapy than to antidepressants alone. Others simply recommend higher-than-usual doses of antidepressants.

ANTIPARKINSONIAN DRUGS

Used for relief of extrapyramidal side effects—adverse reactions resulting from antipsychotic medications.

The earliest and most dramatic reactions are the *acute dystonic reactions.* These occur in the first days of treatment, sometimes after a single dose of medication. They involve bizarre and severe muscle contractions usually of the tongue, face, or extraoccular muscles, producing *torticollis, opisthotonos,* and *occulogyric* crises. These reactions can be physically painful and are almost always frightening to the individual. They are readily reversible with one of the

TABLE 17. ANTIPARKINSONIAN DRUGS*

GENERIC NAME	TRADE NAME	USUAL DOSE
Benztropine	Cogentin	1–2 mg bid† or tid‡
Trihexyphenidyl	Artane	2–5 mg tid or qid§
Biperiden	Akineton	2–4 mg tid or qid
Procyclidine	Kemadrin	5–10 mg tid or qid
Diphenhydramine	Benadryl	25 mg tid or qid

*Source: Adapted from W. S. Appleton and J. M. Davis, *Practical Clinical Psychopharmacology* (Baltimore: Medcom, Inc., 1973), p. 79.© 1973 The Williams & Wilkins Co., Baltimore.

†Twice daily.
‡Three times daily.
§Four times daily.

antiparkinsonian agents—benztropine, 1–2 mg, or diphenhydramine, 25–50 mg intravenously (for immediate relief), intramuscularly (for rapid action), or orally (for relief within hours).

The *parkinsonian syndrome*, named because of its striking resemblance to true Parkinson's disease, commonly occurs after a week or two of the therapy. The hallmark signs include masklike faces, resting tremor, general rigidity of posture with slow voluntary movement, and a shuffling gait. This syndrome, too, is treatable with the antiparkinsonian agents. Oral medication is usually sufficient, since urgency is seldom a consideration in the management of the syndrome.

A third reversible extrapyramidal syndrome is known as *akathisia*. This characteristically is a motor restlessness perceived subjectively by the client and experienced as an urge to pace, a need to shift weight from one foot to another, or an inability to sit or stand still. Generally akathisia is a later complication of drug treatment, occurring weeks to months into the

| | Preparation | |
TABLET	ELIXIR	INJECTABLE
Yes	No	Yes
Yes	Yes	No
Yes	No	Yes
Yes	No	No
Yes	Yes	Yes

course of therapy. Nonetheless, it responds to oral antiparkinsonian agents as well. Accurate observation is essential for akathisia may mimic the symptoms of a psychotic relapse. This interpretation leads to an increase in the dosage of the antipsychotic medication, thus worsening the syndrome.

ANTIPSYCHOTIC DRUGS

This group of drugs affects manifestations of disintegrative patterns including: delusional thinking, confusion, motor agitation, and motor retardation. In addition, antipsychotic drug treatment causes a decrease in formal thought disorder, blunted affect, bizarre behavior, social withdrawal, hallucinations, belligerence, and uncooperativeness. The most common disintegrative condition treated with antipsychotic drugs is the group of symptoms traditionally labeled schizophrenia.

Choice of Specific Drug Controlled studies have failed to demonstrate substantially different antipsychotic effects among these drugs. The choice of a particular medication, then, usually depends on knowledge of the various pharmacologic properties and side effects, the client's or a family member's history of drug response, and the psychiatrist's experience with various compounds. Important client variables are past successes with specific drugs, history of allergies, and history of serious or intolerable side effects.

The principles that govern antipsychotic drug use today are:

- The drugs are given to treat target symptoms of schizophrenia or other psychotic disorders.
- Initial treatment may require parenteral doses. These are changed to oral pill or concentrate forms as the behavior disturbance subsides.
- Total dosages are tailored to individual needs; wide variations exist among clients.
- Divided doses are changed to a single dose primarily at bedtime, as soon as is practical, to maximize use of the drug's sedative properties.
- Most clients with a chronic course require maintenance doses for sustained improvement.

The phenothiazine fluphenazine (Prolixin) is available in long-acting intramuscular injectable forms that behave like sustained-release capsules. The medication is gradually released over a long period of time—2 to 3 weeks. Long-acting Prolixin is available in an enanthate or a decanoate preparation, the difference being that the vehicle substance of the decanoate type releases the medication even more slowly than the enanthate. The main advantages of the long-acting injectable forms are that they largely circumvent a client's ambivalence about taking medication and eliminate the need for constant pill taking.

Use in Certain Age Groups   In elderly persons, the agitation often associated with Organic Mental Syndromes is markedly responsive to phenothiazines. Other sedatives, such as the barbiturates and the benzodiazepines, may further compromise cerebral functioning (further depress the level of awareness and concentration), and thus worsen such syndromes. Doses of phenothizines are generally reduced for the geriatric population,

Antipsychotic medications are effective in treating childhood psychoses and in managing the behavior problems associated with mental retardation. The general principle of reduced dosage is again applicable.

Side Effects

The side effects of antipsychotic medications that nurses must recognize can be divided into the following general classes:

- Autonomic nervous system
- Extrapyramidal
- Other central nervous system
- Allergic
- Blood
- Skin
- Eye
- Endocrine

AUTONOMIC NERVOUS SYSTEM EFFECTS

Anticholinergic side effects include:

Dry mouth

Blurred vision

Constipation

Urinary hesitance or retention

Paralytic ileus (rarer)

Dry mouth symptoms may be relieved by rinsing the mouth with water, chewing sugarless gum, or eating sugarless candy.

A common antiadrenergic effect is postural hypotension. The primary danger is injury from a fall. Blood pressure should be monitored carefully, and clients should be advised to rise from a supine position gradually. Support stockings may be indicated. This problem is more significant when medication is given parenterally.

EXTRAPYRAMIDAL EFFECTS

Acute dystonic reactions

Parkinsonian syndrome

Akathisia

Tardive dyskinesia

The first three extrapyramidal effects are treatable with antiparkinsonian medications. The last syndrome is the most serious since it can be largely irreversible. Tardive dyskinesia is a disorder characterized by involuntary movements of the face, jaw, and tongue resulting in bizarre grimacing, lip smacking and protrusion of the tongue. In addition, there may be jerky choreiform movements of the upper extremities, slow writhing athetoid movements of the arms and the legs, and tense, tonic contractions of the neck and back. The syndrome frequently comes on after years of antipsychotic drug treatment although it can occur earlier. It usually occurs after a maintenance dose is discontinued or reduced, and it can be masked—but not treated—by reinstituting the medication or dosage or by switching to another drug. There is no known cure for the syndrome. The recommended intervention is to stop all medication to see if the syndrome will spontaneously remit.

OTHER CENTRAL NERVOUS SYSTEM EFFECTS

These include sedation and reduction of the seizure threshold. The sedative effects can often be managed by changing to a less sedating agent. Seizures are not a contraindication for the drugs, but they do require close patient observation.

ALLERGIC EFFECTS

The principal allergic manifestation of the antipsychotics is cholestatic jaundice, which arises with chlorpromazine treatment. This occurs much less commonly than it did in the early days of psychopharmacology, and it is usually a benign and self-limited condition.

BLOOD, SKIN, AND EYE EFFECTS

Among the other side effects, *agranulocytosis* (a marked decrease in granulated white blood cells, or leukocytes) is the most serious. It is both potentially fatal and, fortunately, extremely rare. Usually the person gets an infection and deteriorates rapidly or begins to bleed spontaneously. It requires emergency medical attention. Skin eruptions, photosensitivity leading to severe sunburn, blue-grey metallic discolorations over face and hands, and pigmentary changes in the eyes are all potential side effects from chlorpromazine. Clients are generally advised to avoid prolonged exposure to sunlight or to use a sunscreen agent such as sulisobenzone (Uval) when out of doors. These conditions usually remit. One serious eye change that is permanent is retinitis pigmentosa, which may occur in persons on doses of thioridazine exceeding 800 mg per day. This reaction may lead to blindness. Therefore doses exceeding 800 mg per day are contraindicated.

ENDOCRINE EFFECTS

Lactation in females and gynecomastia and impotence in males lead a list of endocrine changes that can occur with antipsychotic drug treatments. The nurse should be alerted to any changes in body function reported.

TABLE 18. SIDE EFFECTS OF COMMONLY USED ANTIPSYCHOTIC MEDICATIONS

CLASS	GENERIC NAME	TRADE NAME	POTENCY (mg EQUIVALENT TO 100 mg CHLORPRO-MAZINE)
Phenothia-zines			
Aliphatic	Chlorprom-azine	Thora-zine	100
Piperadine	Thioridazine	Mellaril	100
Piperizine	Trifluopera-zine	Stela-zine	5
	Fluphena-zine	Prolixin	2
	Perphena-zine	Trilafon	10
Butyrophe-nones	Haloperidol	Haldol	2.5
Thiox-anthenes	Thiothixene	Navane	5
	Chlorpro-thixene	Tarac-tan	100
Dihydro-indolones	Molindone	Moban	10
Dibenzo-xazepines	Loxipine	Loxi-tane	20

**TABLE 19. COMPARATIVE SIDE EFFECTS
OF COMMONLY USED ANTIPSYCHOTIC DRUGS**

EFFECT	CHLORPRO-MAZINE (THORAZINE)	HALO-PERIDOL (HALDOL)	LOXIPINE (LOXITANE)
Akathisia	Occasional	Frequent	Occasional
Allergic skin reactions	Occasional	Rare	Rare

USUAL DOSAGE RANGE mg/DAY	SIDE EFFECTS		
	SEDATIVE	EXTRAPYRAMIDAL	ANTICHOLINERGIC
150–1500	Very strong	Moderate	Strong
150–800	Moderate	Minimal	Moderate
10–60	Weak	Strong	Weak
3–45	Weak	Strong	Weak
12–60	Weak	Strong	Weak
2–40	Weak	Strong	Weak
10–60	Weak	Strong	Weak
40–600	Strong	Moderate	Strong
15–225	Weak	Moderate	Weak
10–100	Moderate	Strong	Moderate

MOLIN-DONE (MOBAN)	THIORI-DAZINE (MELLARIL)	THIO-THIXINE (NAVANE)	TRIFLUO-PERAZINE (STELAZINE)
Frequent	Occasional	Occasional	Frequent
Rare	Not reported	Rare	Rare

(continued)

**TABLE 19. COMPARATIVE SIDE EFFECTS
OF COMMONLY USED ANTIPSYCHOTIC DRUGS (Continued)**

EFFECT	CHLORPRO-MAZINE (THORAZINE)	HALO-PERIDOL (HALDOL)	LOXIPINE (LOXITANE)
Anticho-linergic effects	Frequent	Not reported	Rare
Blood dyscrasia	Occasional	Occasional	Not reported
Cholesta-tic jaundice	Occasional	Rare	Not reported
Dystonias	Occasional	Frequent	Rare
Impotence	Occasional	Not reported	Not reported
Parkin-sonism	Occasional	Frequent	Frequent
Photosen-sitivity	Occasional	Rare	Not reported
Postural hypoten-sion	Frequent	Occasional	Rare
Retinitis pigmen-tosa	Not reported	Not reported	Not reported
Sedation	Frequent	Not reported	Occasional

MOLIN-DONE (MOBAN)	THIORI-DAZINE (MELLARIL)	THIO-THIXINE (NAVANE)	TRIFLUO-PERAZINE (STELAZINE)
Occasional	Frequent	Occasional	Frequent
Rare	Rare	Rare	Rare
Not reported	Rare	Rare	Rare
Occasional	Occasional	Occasional	Frequent
Not reported	Occasional	Not reported	Occasional
Occasional	Occasional	Occasional	Frequent
Not reported	Occasional	Rare	Occasional
Rare	Frequent	Occasional	Rare
Not reported	Occasional	Not reported	Not reported
Rare	Frequent	Frequent	Not reported

Effect of Antipsychotics Used with Other Drugs*

AGENT	EFFECT
Alcohol and/or barbiturates	Speeds action of liver microsomal enzymes so

AGENT	EFFECT
(Alcohol/barbiturates, *continued*)	antipsychotic is metabolized more quickly; potentiates central nervous system depressant effect
Tricyclic antidepressants	Can lead to severe anticholinergic side effects; antipsychotics can raise the plasma level of the antidepressant, probably by inhibiting metabolism of the antidepressant
Hydrochlorthiazide and hydralazine	Can produce severe hypotension
Guanethidine	Antihypertensive effect is blocked by chlorpromazine, haloperidol, and thiothixene
Cigarettes	Heavy consumption requires larger doses of antipsychotic
Meperidine	Respiratory depression is enhanced by chlorpromazine
Anticonvulsants	Seizure threshold may be lowered by antipsychotic requiring adjustment of anticonvulsant
Levodopa	Antiparkinsonian effect may be inhibited by antipsychotics

AGENT	EFFECT
General anesthesia	Antipsychotic may potentiate effect of anesthetic

*Source: From material by E. Harris, copyright © 1981, American Journal of Nursing Company. Reproduced with permission from *The American Journal of Nursing*, Vol. 81, No. 7 (July 1981).

Drug Information Card for Antipsychotic Agents (Health Teaching)

ANTIPSYCHOTICS (Thorazine, Mellaril, Stelazine, Prolixin, Trilafon, Haldol, Navane, Moban, Loxitane)

Action: This medication will help you to relax, think more clearly, and keep your thoughts together.

Side Effects/Precautions:

1. You may experience drowsiness, blurred vision, dry mouth, or constipation while taking this medication.
2. Do not use alcohol or other depressant drugs while taking this medication. Any use of alcohol or other drugs should be discussed with your doctor.
3. Do not drive a car until you are sure the medication does not make you drowsy.
4. You may experience dizziness or lightheadedness. Get up from a lying position slowly, as standing quickly can cause dizziness. In the morning when you awaken, sit up in the bed for one full minute before standing.
5. If you develop a sore throat without other cold or flu symptoms, this should be reported to your doctor.
6. You may experience periods of muscle stiffening or

muscle restlessness. These symptoms should be reported to your doctor.

7. Your skin may be extremely sensitive to the sun. If you are going to be outside, be sure your skin is covered or use a sun-screening preparatrion containing para amino benzoic acid (PABA). The following products contain PABA: Pabanol (Elder Company), Pre Sun (Eastwood Pharmaceuticals).

8. This medication may rarely cause females to miss menstrual periods. If this occurs, notify your doctor.

9. It is important to take this medication exactly as directed by your doctor. Do not stop taking the medication or change the dosage without contacting your doctor. If you forget a dose during the day, you may take that dose later in the day.

10. Notify your doctor if you are constipated or have difficulty passing urine. Use of a stool softener such as dioctyl sodium sulfosuccinate, or Colace, may be beneficial if you are constipated.

11. Do not take antacids (Maalox, Mylanta, etc.) within an hour of taking this medication.

Your drug is _____

Your dosage is _____

Adapted from Smith, J. E., April 1981, Improving Drug Knowledge in Psychiatric Patients. *Journal of Psychiatric Nursing and Mental Health Services.*

HYPNOTIC DRUGS

Many of the hypnotic drugs tend to have undesirable effects, including physiologic addiction, fatal overdose potential and dangerous interactions with other medications because of liver enzyme induction. The first principle of treatment is to assess whether the insomnia is related to one of the major mental disorders, such as schizophrenia or major depression. If so, the insomnia can and should be treated as part of the larger problem, and sedative antipsychotics or antidepressants may be given at bedtime to accomplish this purpose.

Benzodiazepines

In the management of simple insomnia without an associated mental disorder, a benzodiazepine compound flurazepam (Dalmane), 15 mg or 30 mg at bedtime, is the drug of choice. This drug is generally both effective and safe; it is the one sleeping medication that does not interfere with rapid eye movement (REM) during sleep and therefore can be used on consecutive nights for approximately a month.

Barbiturates

Commonly prescribed for their hypnotic effects, their only advantage over the benzodiazepines is their low cost. Barbiturates, especially the short-acting types, such as secobarbital (Seconal), are powerfully addicting substances. They are frequently used in successful suicide attempts because overdoses can cause severe central nervous system respiratory depression. Barbiturates suppress REM sleep, leading to the phenomenon of REM deprivation and REM rebound—that is, after a week or two of treatment, they help create the insomnia they were intended to control. Barbiturates also speed up the metabolism of anticoagulant and other drugs because they induce liver enzyme synthesis. This effect can be fatal. Long-acting barbiturates (phenobarbital) are very useful, however, in the detoxification of barbiturate addicts and the management of epilepsy.

Other Insomnia Drugs

Several nonbarbiturate hypnotics are also of questionable value. Among these are ethchlorvynol (Placidyl), which is fatal in doses only five times the usual therapeutic dose, and glutethimide (Doriden), which is addicting and produces complicated, fluctuating, and difficult-to-manage states of consciousness following overdose. There seem to be no valid indications for the use of these two drugs. Chloral hydrate (Noctec) and methyprylon (Noludar) can be used under closely controlled conditions such as those in an inpatient psychiatric service. (See Table 20, page 366.)

LITHIUM (ANTIMANIA DRUG)

Many well-controlled studies indicate unequivocally that lithium is the most effective agent for treating the vast majority of acute manic and hypomanic episodes. In addition, because of the absence of sedative side effects, the client feels much more related to the environment and able to function normally while under the influence of lithium. An accurate diagnosis of mania is, as always, the most important factor in maximizing the effect of positive clinical response.

Dosage The management of an acute manic episode involves rapid initiation of lithium, increased to substantial doses during the first week of treatment. Usually between 1500 and 2100 mg per day are needed by the average-sized client in an acute period. Lithium is available only in oral form in 250-mg and 300-mg capsules and tablets. Since lithium is an ion, its concentration can be measured in the blood. In the acute phase the blood level usually must attain a concentration of 1.0-1.5 mEq/L. After a week to 10 days, as the symptoms subside, the dose can be decreased to 900–1200 mg per day, with the blood level maintained in the range of 0.7-1.2 mEq/L for continuing control.

The basic principles for antimania drug therapy are:

- Lithium is indicated and effective in the treatment of acute manic episodes and in the prevention of recurrent manic or depressive episodes.
- Lithium is given in divided doses with increases in the daily dose until the blood level reaches 1.0-1.5 mEq/L in acute states of the disorder. Blood levels must be monitored after each increase.
- Antipsychotic medications may be necessary early in the course of treatment for behavior control.
- Following symptom resolution, lithium is decreased for maintenance treatment to approximately one-half to two-thirds the acute dose. Blood levels are checked every 2-3 months or when there is reason to suspect a change.

Side Effects Lithium has a significant number of side effects that can be troublesome and, in some cases, quite dangerous. Significant side effects are usually correlated with blood levels above 1.5 mEq/L. Common side effects include tremor, nausea, thirst, and polyuria; thyroid goiter has also been seen. Severe lithium poisoning presents a potential medical emergency. Early signs include vomiting and diarrhea, lethargy, and muscle twitching. These may progress to ataxia and slurred speech. A serious situation exists when the client becomes semiconscious or comatose. At that point seizures may occur, and electrolyte imbalances may lead to cardiac arrest. This syndrome of severe toxicity ordinarily occurs only when the client has a lithium level of 2.0-3.0 mEq/L. The client may have overdosed or severely restricted food or salt intake (or taken diuretics) to induce this state.

(Text continues on page 369.)

TABLE 20. SIDE EFFECTS OF HYPNOTIC AGENTS*

CLASS	GENERIC NAME	TRADE NAME	USUAL DOSAGE RANGE (mg AT BEDTIME)	REM SLEEP DEPRESSION	LIVER ENZYME INDUCTION	ADDICTIVE POTENTIAL
					SIDE EFFECTS	
Benzodiazepines	Flurazepam	Dalmane	15–30	No	No	Lower
Barbiturates (short-acting)	Secobarbital	Seconal	100	Yes	Yes	Higher
	Pentobarbital	Nembutal	100–200	Yes	Yes	Higher
Chloral derivatives	Chloral hydrate	Noctec	500–1000	Probable	No	Higher
Others	Methyprylon	Noludar	200–400	Yes	?	Higher
	Glutethimide	Doriden	500–1000	Yes	Yes	Higher
	Ethchlorvynol	Placidyl	500–1000	?	?	Higher
	Methaqualone	Quaalude	150–400	Probable	?	Higher

*Source: Compiled from Shader, R. T. 1975. *Manual of Psychiatric Therapeutics*. Boston: Little, Brown and Co. pp. 312–315.

TABLE 21. ADDICTIVE DOSES OF SEDATIVE HYPNOTICS*

GENERIC NAME	TRADE NAME	DEPENDENCE-PRODUCING DOSE (mg PER DAY)	NUMBER OF DAYS NECESSARY TO PRODUCE DEPENDENCE
Chloridiazepoxide	Librium	300–600	60–180
Diazepam	Valium	80–120	42
Chloral hydrate	Noctec	2000–3000	
Meprobamate	Equanil		
	Miltown		
Glutethimide	Doriden	200–3000	
Sodium secobarbital	Seconal	800–2200	35–37
Sodium pentobarbital	Nembutal	800–2200	35–37
Methaqualone	Sopor	2100–3000	21–28
	Quaalude		

*Source: Reprinted with permission of STASH, Inc. from the *Journal of Psychedelic Drugs*, Volume 3(2):81, Spring, 1971. Copyright © 1971.

TABLE 22. SIDE EFFECTS FROM LITHIUM CARBONATE THERAPY*

ORGAN SYSTEM AFFECTED	MILD (NORMAL)	MODERATE (MAY BE NORMAL OR MAY SUGGEST IMPENDING TOXICITY)	SEVERE (TOXIC)	EXTREME
Gastrointestinal tract	Nausea	Anorexia, vomiting, diarrhea, thirst	None	None
Neuromuscular system	Tremor	Muscle weakness, muscle hyperirritability, coarse tremor, ataxia	Hypertonic muscles, hyperactive reflexes, choreoathetoid movements	None
Central nervous system	None	Sedation, fatigue, giddiness	Blurred vision, slurred speech, vertigo, somnolence, confusion, stupor, local neurologic signs, seizures	Coma Death
Cardiovascular system	None	None	Pulse irregularities, hypotension, electro-cardiogram abnormalties	Circulatory collapse
Miscellaneous	None	Polyuria, glycosuria, dehydration	None	None

Source: Compiled from Klein, D. F. and Davis, J. M. 1964. *Diagnosis and Drug Treatment of Psychiatric Disorders.* Baltimore: Williams and Wilkins Co., p. 238; and Shader, R. I. 1975. *Manual of Psychiatric Therapeutics* Boston: Little, Brown and Co. p. 110.

Drug Information Card for Lithium Carbonate (Health Teaching)

LITHIUM CARBONATE (Eskalith, Lithane)

Action: This medication maintains an even mood. It is used to treat bipolar disorder and to prevent recurrent depressions.

Side Effects/Precautions:

1. Take this medication *exactly* as directed by your doctor. You must take the medication every day at the indicated time (e.g., morning and evening; morning, noon, and evening, etc.). If you skip a dose, *do not* double the dosage the next time you take your medication, but continue your regular schedule.
2. Be sure to maintain an adequate fluid intake, since you may urinate more than usual.
3. Do not take any other medication, including over-the-counter products, without consulting your M.D. or pharmacist. Do not take a diuretic (water pill) unless directed to do so by your doctor. Be sure to tell any other doctor that you visit that you are taking lithium.
4. It is important to maintain a normal, well-balanced diet while taking this medication. Be sure you do not become dehydrated by excessive heat or exercise. If you do sweat a great deal because of heat or exercise, you should try to replace some of the salt you have lost by eating a salty snack like pretzels or potato chips. You may also take salt tablets if approved by your doctor.
5. When you first start taking this medication, you may experience excessive urination, mild nausea, or general discomfort. These symptoms will pass in a few weeks. If they persist, contact your doctor.
6. Contact your doctor if you have any of the following

(Text continues on page 374.)

TABLE 23. A NURSING CARE PLAN FOR CLIENTS ON LITHIUM*

PROBLEM	OBJECTIVE	NURSING INTERVENTIONS
Air, Food, Fluid		
Intake of food and fluid is impaired by side effects affecting the gastrointestinal (GI) system.	To maintain balanced food and fluid intake	Obtain diet history to determine usual intake. Monitor intake of foods containing sodium. Teach clients to avoid fluctuations of sodium intake. Monitor fluid intake. Encourage at least six to eight glasses fluid per day.
	To support clients when they experience unavoidable side effects	Administer lithium spaced through the day three or four times daily. Give with meals or with food in the stomach. Give tea and crackers for nausea. Teach clients to rinse mouth frequently and practice oral hygiene when they experience dryness of the mouth.

Elimination

Bowel and urinary elimination is altered by side effects affecting the gastrointestinal system and kidney functioning.

To maintain balanced intake and output

To support clients when they experience unavoidable side effects

Monitor bowel and bladder output.

Observe for persistence and exacerbations of GI side effects.

Personal Hygiene and Body Temperature

Physical hygiene needs and maintenance may be altered by side effects.

To promote and maintain physical hygiene and skin integrity

Assess skin condition and hygiene needs.

Monitor symptoms of edema through measuring extremities with a tape measure.

Teach clients to elevate legs when edema is present.

Teach and assist clients to perform routine personal hygiene.

Monitor skin condition and observe for signs of dehydration, pruritus, or hypothyroidism.

Observe for persistence and exacerbations of GI side effects.

TABLE 23. A NURSING CARE PLAN FOR CLIENTS ON LITHIUM Continued

PROBLEM	OBJECTIVE	NURSING INTERVENTIONS
Fluid and electrolyte balance may be altered by changes in body temperature.	Limit alterations in body temperature Promote fluid-electrolyte balance	Assess body temperature. Assist clients to choose clothes appropriate for weather conditions. Teach clients to avoid exposure to extreme fluctuations in climate. Monitor sodium intake.
Rest and Activity Rest and activity may be impaired by side effects affecting various body systems.	To promote a balance of rest and activity To support the client when he experiences unavoidable side effects	Assess rest/activity pattern. Identify activity that may result in excessive perspiration. Protect clients from exhaustion due to overactivity by providing a quiet room and limited stimulation. Promote safety through teaching clients to avoid operating an

automobile or smoking alone if they experience lethargy.
Assist clients to plan schedule for rest and activity.

Solitude and Socialization

Skills needed for solitude and socialization may be impaired by symptoms of the client.

To develop a balance of solitude/socialization patterns and skills

Assist clients to learn the effects and side effects of lithium carbonate.
Assist clients to learn difference between effects, side effects, and symptoms of their illness.

*Source: From "Nursing Care of Patients on Lithium," by Susan Humn, Cecile Miranda, Vivian Molyneaux, and Catherine Warshaw, *Perspectives in Psychiatric Care* Vol. 18, No. 5 (Sept.-Oct., 1980).

symptoms: diarrhea, vomiting, fine tremors of the hands, drowsiness, muscular weakness, or ringing in the ears.

7. Your doctor or pharmacist may give you an identification card which states that you are taking lithium. Carry this with you at all times.

8. On the day that you have your lithium blood level drawn, do not take a dose of lithium for 8–12 hours prior to the blood test.

Your drug is _____

Your dosage is _____

*From drug cards written by Janet E. Smith RN, MSN.

APPENDIX C

SKILLS THAT FOSTER EFFECTIVE COMMUNICATION

GIVING FEEDBACK

Focus feedback on behavior rather than on client.

Focus feedback on observations rather than inferences.

Focus feedback on description rather than judgment.

Focus feedback on "more or less" rather than "either/or" descriptions of behavior.

Focus feedback on here-and-now behavior rather than there-and-then behavior.

Focus feedback on sharing of information and ideas rather than advice.

Focus feedback on exploration of alternatives rather than answers or solutions.

Focus feedback on its value to client rather than on catharsis it provides nurse.

Limit feedback to amount of information client is able to use rather than amount nurse has available to give.

Limit feedback to appropriate time and place.

Focus feedback on what is said rather than why it is said.

REFLECTING

Reflecting can respond to two dimensions of communication—content and feelings. In reflecting the *content* of the message, the nurse repeats basically the same statement as the client. This gives the client the opportunity to hear and mull over what he or she has said:

"You believe things will be better soon."

"You think it would be better to take a part-time job."

Content reflection is perhaps one of the most misused and overused methods in mental health counseling. It loses its effectiveness when used for lack of other choices.

Reflecting *feelings* consists of verbalizing what seems to be implied about feelings in the client's comment.

"Sounds like you're really angry at your brother."

"You're feeling uncomfortable about being discharged from the hospital."

In reflecting feelings, the nurse attempts to identify latent and connotative meanings that may either further clarify or distort the content. Reflection is useful because it encourages the client to make additional clarifying comments.

IMPARTING INFORMATION

Statements that give information help the client by supplying additional data. They therefore encourage further clarification based on new or additional input.

"Group therapy will be held on Tuesday evening from 6:30 until 8:00."

"I am a nursing student."

It is not constructive to withhold helpful or useful information from the client or to reply "What do you think?" to a straightforward information-seeking question. However, the nurse must be careful not to distort the giving of information into advice or use it to avoid an area of interpersonal difficulty. If the nurse gives personal social information, the conversation may move out of the realm of therapeutic intervention.

CLARIFYING

Clarifying is an attempt to understand the basic nature of a client's statement.

"I'm confused about... could you go over that again, please."

"You say you're feeling anxious now. What's that like for you?"

Asking the client to give an example to clarify a meaning helps the nurse to understand the client's intended message better. A person who describes a concrete incident is more likely to be able to see the connections between it and similar occurrences. Illustrations are very useful qualifiers.

PARAPHRASING

In paraphrasing, the nurse restates what she or he has heard the client communicating.

"In other words, you're fed up with being treated like a child."

"I hear you saying that when people compliment you, you feel embarrassed. If they knew the real you, they'd stay away."

Paraphrasing offers the opportunity to test the nurse's understanding of what the client is attempting to communicate. It is reflective in nature, in that it lets the client know how another person is understanding the message.

CHECKING PERCEPTIONS

The nurse who shares how she or he perceives and hears the client is engaged in the process of checking perceptions. After sharing perceptions of the client's behaviors, thoughts, and feelings, the nurse asks the client to verify the perception.

"Let me know if this is how you see it too."

"I get the feeling that you're uncomfortable when we're silent. Does that seem to fit?"

A perception check is used to make sure that the nurse understands the client. An effective perception check conveys the message "I want to understand...." It allows the other person the opportunity to correct inaccurate perceptions. It also allows the nurse to avoid actions based on false assumptions about the client.

PROCESSING

Processing is the most complex and sophisticated technique used by the nurse. Process comments are those that direct attention to the interpersonal dynamics of the nurse-client experience. These dynamics are illustrated in the content, feelings, and behavior expressed.

"It seems that important things that need to be taken care of come up in the last 5 minutes we have together in our session."

"Today is the first day our session has started out with silence. Last week it seemed there wouldn't be enough time."

Processing is most useful when therapeutic intimacy has been achieved.

STRUCTURING

Structuring is an attempt to create order or evolve guidelines. The nurse helps the client to become aware of problems and the order in which they might be dealt with.

"You've mentioned that you want to improve your relationships with your wife, your sister, and your boss. Let's put them in order of priority."

"No, I won't be giving you advice, but we can discuss the possible solutions together."

Structuring is particularly useful when clients introduce a number of concerns in a brief period of time with little idea of which to begin work on. In addition to structuring content, nurses use structuring to delimit the parameters of the nurse-client relationship and identify how the nurse will participate with the client in the problem-solving process.

PINPOINTING

Pinpointing calls attention to certain kinds of statements and relationships. For example, the nurse may point to inconsistencies among statements or to similarities and differences in the points of view, feelings, or actions of two or more persons, or between what one says and what one does.

"So, you and your wife don't agree about how many children you want."

"You say you're sad, but you're smiling."

LINKING

In linking, the nurse responds to the client in a way that ties together two events, experiences, feelings, or persons. Linking may be used to connect past experiences with current behaviors. Another example is linking the tension between two persons with current life stress.

"You felt depressed after the birth of both your children."

"Do you think the trouble is more with him or with you, since you both have been under increased job strain?"

QUESTIONING

Questioning is a very direct way of speaking with clients. But when used to excess, questioning controls the nature and range of the client's responses. Questions can be useful when the nurse is seeking specific information. When the nurse's intent is to engage the client in meaningful dialogue, however, questions should be limited.

When the nurse is using questions, it is best to make them open-ended rather than closed. An *open-ended question* focuses the topic but allows freedom of response.

"How were you feeling when your mother said that to you?"

"What's your opinion about...."

The *closed question* limits the client's choice of responses generally to "yes" or "no" ("Were you feeling angry when your mother said that?"). Closed questions limit therapeutic exploration.

"Why" questions usually have the same effect. They often are impossible to answer and rarely lead to a clearer understanding of the situation. However, "who," "what," "when," and "how" questions may be helpful when used judiciously.

CONFRONTING

There are six skills to be incorporated in constructive confrontations. They are:

1. Use of personal statements with the words *I, my,* and *me*
2. Use of relationship statements in which the nurse expresses what he or she thinks or feels about the client in the interaction
3. Use of behavior descriptions (statements describing the visible behavior of the client)
4. Use of description of personal feelings, specifying the feeling by name
5. Use of responses aimed at understanding, such as paraphrasing and perception checking
6. Use of constructive feedback skills

"When you wring your hands I feel anxious."

"Sometimes when you turn your head away from me I think you're angry."

SUMMARIZING

Summarizing is a way of highlighting the main ideas that have been discussed. It reviews for the client and the nurse what the main themes of the conversation were. Summarizing is also useful in focusing the client's thinking and aiding conscious learning.

"The last time we were together you were concerned about...."

"You had three main concerns today...."

This technique can be used appropriately at different times in the client-nurse interaction. For example, summarizing the previous interaction is useful in the first few minutes of the time the nurse and the client spend together. When summarization occurs early, it helps the client recall the areas discussed and also provides the client with the opportunity to see how the nurse has synthesized the content of a previous session. Summarizing is useful because it keeps the participants directed toward a goal.

APPENDIX D

DSM-III CLASSIFICATION: AXIS I–V

All official DSM-III codes and terms are included in ICD-9-CM. However, in order to differentiate those DSM–III categories that use the same ICD-9-CM codes, unofficial non-ICD-9-CM codes are provided in parentheses for use when greater specificity is necessary.

The long dashes indicate the need for a fifth-digit subtype or other qualifying term.

AXES I AND II: CATEGORIES AND CODES

Disorders Usually First Evident in Infancy, Childhood, or Adolescence

MENTAL RETARDATION

(Code in fifth digit: 1 = with other behavioral symptoms (requiring attention or treatment and that are not part of another disorder), 0 = without other behavioral symptoms.)

317.0(x) Mild Mental Retardation, _____
318.0(x) Moderate Mental Retardation, _____
318.1(x) Severe Mental Retardation, _____
318.2(x) Profound Mental Retardation, _____
319.0(x) Unspecified Mental Retardation, _____

ATTENTION DEFICIT DISORDER

314.01 with Hyperactivity
314.00 without Hyperactivity
314.80 Residual Type

Source: The American Psychiatric Association, Diagnostic and Statistical Manual of Mental Disorders, Third Edition, Washington, D.C., A.P.A. 1980. Reprinted by permission.

CONDUCT DISORDER

312.00 Undersocialized, Aggressive
312.10 Undersocialized, Nonagressive
312.23 Socialized, Aggressive
312.21 Socialized, Nonagressive
312.90 Atypical

ANXIETY DISORDERS OF CHILDHOOD OR ADOLESCENCE

309.21 Separation Anxiety Disorder
313.21 Avoidant Disorder of Childhood or Adolescence
313.99 Overanxious Disorder

OTHER DISORDERS OF INFANCY, CHILDHOOD, OR ADOLESCENCE

313.89 Reactive Attachment Disorder of Infancy
313.22 Schizoid Disorder of Childhood or Adolescence
313.23 Elective Mutism
313.81 Oppositional Disorder
313.82 Identity Disorder

EATING DISORDERS

307.10 Anorexia Nervosa
307.51 Bulimia
307.52 Pica
307.53 Rumination Disorder of Infancy
307.50 Atypical Eating Disorder

STEREOTYPED MOVEMENT DISORDERS

307.21 Transient Tic Disorder
307.22 Chronic Motor Tic Disorder
307.23 Tourette's Disorder
307.20 Atypical Tic Disorder
307.30 Atypical Stereotyped Movement Disorder

OTHER DISORDERS WITH PHYSICAL MANIFESTATIONS

307.00 Stuttering
307.60 Functional Enuresis

384

307.70 Functional Encopresis
307.46 Sleepwalking Disorder
307.46 Sleep Terror Disorder (307.49)

PERVASIVE DEVELOPMENTAL DISORDERS

Code in fifth digit: 0 = Full Syndrome Present, 1 = Residual State.

299.0x Infantile Autism, ____
299.9x Childhood Onset Pervasive Developmental Disorder, ____
299.8x Atypical, ____

SPECIFIC DEVELOPMENTAL DISORDERS

Note: These are coded on Axis II.

315.00 Developmental Reading Disorder
315.10 Developmental Arithmetic Disorder
315.31 Developmental Language Disorder
315.39 Developmental Articulation Disorder
315.50 Mixed Specific Developmental Disorder
315.90 Atypical Specific Developmental Disorder

Organic Mental Disorders

Section 1. Organic Mental Disorders whose etiology or pathophysiological process is listed on page 386 (taken from the mental disorders section of ICD-9-CM).

DEMENTIAS ARISING IN THE SENIUM AND PRESENIUM

Primary Degenerative Dementia, Senile Onset,
290.30 with Delirium
290.20 with Delusions
290.21 with Depression
290.00 Uncomplicated

Code in fifth digit:
1 = with Delirium, 2 = with Delusions, 3 = with Depression, 0 = Uncomplicated.
290.1x Primary Degenerative Dementia, Presenile Onset, ____
290.4x Multi-infarct Dementia, ____

SUBSTANCE-INDUCED

Alcohol
303.00 Intoxication
291.40 Idiosyncratic Intoxication
291.80 Withdrawal
291.00 Withdrawal Delirium
291.30 Hallucinosis
291.10 Amnestic Disorder
Code severity of Dementia in fifth Digit: 1 = Mild, 2 = Moderate, 3 = Severe, 0 = Unspecified.
291.2x Dementia Associated with Alcoholism, ____

Barbiturate or similarly acting sedative or hypnotic
305.40 Intoxication (327.00)
292.00 Withdrawal (327.01)
292.00 Withdrawal Delirium (327.02)
292.83 Amnestic Disorder (327.04)

Opioid
305.50 Intoxication (327.10)
292.00 Withdrawal (327.11)

Cocaine
305.60 Intoxication (327.20)

Amphetamine or similarly acting sympathomimetic
305.70 Intoxication (327.30)
292.81 Delirium (327.32)
292.11 Delusional Disorder (327.35)
292.00 Withdrawal (327.31)

Phencyclidine (PCP) or similarly acting
Arylcyclohexylamine

305.90 Intoxication (327.40)
292.81 Delirium (327.42)
292.90 Mixed Organic Mental Disorder (327.49)

Hallucinogen
305.30 Hallucinosis (327.56)
292.11 Delusional Disorder (327.55)
292.84 Affective Disorder (327.57)

Cannabis
305.20 Intoxication (327.60)
292.11 Delusional Disorder (327.65)

Tobacco
292.00 Withdrawal (327.71)

Caffeine
305.90 Intoxication (327.80)

Other or Unspecified Substance
305.90 Intoxication (327.90)
292.00 Withdrawal (327.91)
292.81 Delirium (327.92)
292.82 Dementia (327.93)
292.83 Amnestic Disorder (327.94)
292.11 Delusional Disorder (327.95)
292.12 Hallucinosis (327.96)
292.84 Affective Disorder (327.97)
292.89 Personality Disorder (327.98)
292.90 Atypical or Mixed Organic Mental Disorder
       (327.99)

Section 2.   Organic Brain Syndromes whose etiology or pathophysiological process is either noted as an additional diagnosis from outside the mental disorders section of ICD-9-CM or is unknown.

293.00 Delirium
294.10 Dementia
294.00 Amnestic Syndrome
293.81 Organic Delusional Syndrome

293.82 Organic Hallucinosis
293.83 Organic Affective Syndrome
310.10 Organic Personality Syndrome
294.80 Atypical or Mixed Organic Brain Syndrome

Substance Use Disorders

Code in fifth digit: 1 = Continuous, 2 = Episodic, 3 = in Remission, 0 = Unspecified

305.0x Alcohol Abuse, ____
303.9x Alcohol Dependence (Alcoholism), ____
305.4x Barbiturate or similarly acting sedative or hypnotic Abuse, ____
304.1x Barbiturate or similarly acting sedative or hypnotic Dependence, ____
305.5x Opioid Abuse, ____
304.0x Opioid Dependence, ____
305.6x Cocaine Abuse, ____
305.7x Amphetamine or similarly acting sympath-omimetic Abuse, ____
304.4x Amphetamine or similarly acting sympatho-mimetic Dependence, ____
305.9x Phencyclidine (PCP) or similarly acting arylcyclohexylamine Abuse, ____ (328.4x)
305.3x Hallucinogen Abuse, ____
305.2x Cannabis Abuse, ____
304.3x Cannabis Dependence, ____
305.1x Tobacco Dependence, ____
305.9x Other, mixed or unspecified Substance Abuse, ____
304.6x Other Specified Substance Dependence, ____
304.9x Unspecified Substance Dependence, ____
304.7x Dependence on Combination of Opiod and other Nonalcoholic Substance, ____
304.8x Dependence on Combination of Substances, excluding opioids and alcohol, ____

Schizophrenic Disorders

Code in fifth digit: 1 = Subchronic, 2 = Chronic, 3 = Subchronic with Acute Exacerbation, 4 = Chronic with Acute Exacerbation, 5 = in Remission, 0 = Unspecified.

Schizophrenia
295.1x Disorganized, _____
295.2x Catatonic, _____
295.3x Paranoid, _____
295.9x Undifferentiated, _____
295.6x Residual, _____

Paranoid Disorders

297.10 Paranoia
297.30 Shared Paranoid Disorder
298.30 Acute Paranoid Disorder
297.90 Atypical Paranoid Disorder

Psychotic Disorders Not Elsewhere Classified

295.40 Schizophreniform Disorder
298.80 Brief Reactive Psychosis
295.70 Schizoaffective Disorder
298.90 Atypical Psychosis

Neurotic Disorders

These are included in Affective, Anxiety, Somatoform, Dissociative, and Psychosexual Disorders. In order to facilitate the identification of the categories that in DSM II were grouped together in the class of Neuroses, the DSM-II terms are included separately in parentheses after the corresponding categories. These DSM-II terms are included in ICD-9-CM and therefore are acceptable as alternatives to the recommended DSM-III terms that precede them.

Affective Disorders

MAJOR AFFECTIVE DISORDERS

Code Major Depressive Episode in fifth digit: 6 = in Remission, 4 = with Psychotic Features (the unofficial non-ICD-9-CM fifth digit 7 may be used instead to indicate that the psychotic features are mood-incongruent), 3 = with Melancholia, 2 = without Melancholia, 0 = Unspecified.

Code Manic Episode in fifth digit: 6 = in Remission, 4 = with Psychotic Features (the unofficial non-ICD-9-CM fifth digit 7 may be used instead to indicate that the psychotic features are mood-incongruent), 2 = without Psychotic Features, 0 = Unspecified.

Bipolar Disorder
296.6x Mixed, ____
296.4x Manic, ____
296.5x Depressed, ____

Major Depression
296.2x Single Episode, ____
296.3x Recurrent, ____

OTHER SPECIFIC AFFECTIVE DISORDERS

301.13 Cyclothymic Disorder
300.40 Dysthymic Disorder (or Depressive Neurosis)

ATYPICAL AFFECTIVE DISORDERS

296.70 Atypical Bipolar Disorder
296.82 Atypical Depression

Anxiety Disorders

PHOBIC DISORDERS (OR PHOBIC NEUROSES)

300.21 Agoraphobia with Panic Attacks
300.22 Agoraphobia without Panic Attacks
300.23 Social Phobia
300.29 Simple Phobia

ANXIETY STATES (OR ANXIETY NEUROSES)

300.01 Panic Disorder
300.02 Generalized Anxiety Disorder
300.30 Obsessive Compulsive Disorder (or Obsessive
          Compulsive Neurosis)

POST-TRAUMATIC STRESS DISORDER

308.30 Acute
309.81 Chronic or Delayed
300.00 Atypical Anxiety Disorder

Somatoform Disorders

300.81 Somatization Disorder
300.11 Conversion Disorder (or Hysterical Neurosis,
          Conversion Type)
307.80 Psychogenic Pain Disorder
300.70 Hypochondriasis (or Hypochondriacal
          Neurosis)
300.70 Atypical Somatoform Disorder (300.71)

Dissociative Disorders (or Hysterical Neuroses, Dissociative Type)

300.12 Psychogenic Amnesia
300.13 Psychogenic Fugue
300.14 Multiple Personality
300.60 Depersonalization Disorder (or
          Depersonalization Neurosis)
300.15 Atypical Dissociative Disorder

Psychosexual Disorders

GENDER IDENTITY DISORDERS

Indicate sexual history in the fifth digit of Transsexualism code: 1 = Asexual, 2 = Homosexual, 3 = Heterosexual, 0 = Unspecified.
302.5x Transsexualism, ____
302.60 Gender Identity Disorder of Childhood
302.85 Atypical Gender Identity Disorder

PARAPHILIAS

302.81 Fetishism
302.30 Transvestism
302.10 Zoophilia
302.20 Pedophilia
302.40 Exhibitionism
302.82 Voyeurism
302.83 Sexual Masochism
302.84 Sexual Sadism
302.90 Atypical Paraphilia

PSYCHOSEXUAL DYSFUNCTIONS

302.71 Inhibited Sexual Desire
302.72 Inhibited Sexual Excitement
302.73 Inhibited Female Orgasm
302.74 Inhibited Male Orgasm
302.75 Premature Ejaculation
302.76 Functional Dyspareunia
306.51 Functional Vaginismus
302.70 Atypical Psychosexual Dysfunction

OTHER PSYCHOSEXUAL DISORDERS

302.00 Ego-dystonic Homosexuality
302.89 Psychosexual Disorder not elsewhere classified

Factitious Disorders

300.16 Factitious Disorder with Psychological
        Symptoms
301.51 Chronic Factitious Disorder with Physical
        Symptoms
300.19 Atypical Factitious Disorder with Physical
        Symptoms

Disorders of Impulse Control Not Elsewhere Classified

312.31 Pathological Gambling
312.32 Kleptomania
312.33 Pyromania

392

312.34 Intermittent Explosive Disorder
312.35 Isolated Explosive Disorder
312.39 Atypical Impulse Control Disorder

Adjustment Disorder

309.00 with Depressed Mood
309.24 with Anxious Mood
309.28 with Mixed Emotional Features
309.30 with Disturbance of Conduct
309.40 with Mixed Disturbance of Emotions and
Conduct
309.23 with Work (or Academic) Inhibition
309.83 with Withdrawal
309.90 with Atypical Features

Psychological Factors Affecting Physical Condition

Specify physical condition on Axis III.
316.00 Psychological Factors Affecting Physical
Condition

PERSONALITY DISORDERS

Note: These are coded on Axis II.

301.00 Paranoid
301.20 Schizoid
301.22 Schizotypal
301.50 Histrionic
301.81 Narcissistic
301.70 Antisocial
301.83 Borderline
301.82 Avoidant
301.60 Dependent
301.40 Compulsive
301.84 Passive-Aggressive
301.89 Atypical, Mixed or other
Personality Disorder

V Codes for Conditions Not Attributable to a Mental Disorder That Are a Focus of Attention or Treatment

V65.20 Malingering
V62.89 Borderline Intellectual Functioning (V62.88)
V71.01 Adult Antisocial Behavior
V71.02 Childhood or Adolescent Antisocial Behavior
V62.30 Academic Problem
V62.20 Occupational Problem
V62.82 Uncomplicated Bereavement
V15.81 Noncompliance with Medical Treatment
V62.89 Phase of Life Problem or Other Life
        Circumstance Problem
V61.10 Marital Problem
V61.20 Parent-child Problem
V61.80 Other Specified Family Circumstances
V62.81 Other Interpersonal Problem

Additional Codes

300.90 Unspecified Mental Disorder (Nonpsychotic)
V71.09 No Diagnosis or Condition on Axis I
799.90 Diagnosis or Condition Deferred on Axis I

V71.09 No Diagnosis on Axis II
799.90 Diagnosis Deferred on Axis II

AXIS III: PHYSICAL DISORDERS OR CONDITIONS

Axis III permits the clinician to indicate any current physical disorder or condition that is potentially relevant to the understanding or management of the client. These are the conditions exclusive of the "mental disorders section" of ICD-9-CM. (The 9th edition of the International Classification of Diseases.) In some instances the condition may be etiologically significant; in other instances the physical disorder is important to the overall management of the client. In yet other instances, the clinician may wish to note the presence of other significant associated physical assessment findings, such as "soft neurological signs." Multiple diagnoses are permitted on this axis.

AXIS IV: SEVERITY OF PSYCHOSOCIAL STRESSORS

CODE	TERM	ADULT EXAMPLES	CHILD OR ADOLESCENT EXAMPLES
1	None	No apparent psychosocial stressor	No apparent psychosocial stressor
2	Minimal	Minor violation of the law; small bank loan	Vacation with family
3	Mild	Argument with neighbor; change in work hours	Change in schoolteacher; new school year
4	Moderate	New career; death of close friend; pregnancy	Chronic parental fighting; change to new school; illness of close relative; birth of sibling
5	Severe	Serious illness in self or family; major financial loss; marital separation; birth of child	Death of peer; divorce of parents; arrest; hospitalization; persistent and harsh parental discipline
6	Extreme	Death of close relative; divorce	Death of parent or sibling;

CODE	TERM	ADULT EXAMPLES	CHILD OR ADOLESCENT EXAMPLES
			repeated physical or sexual abuse
7	Catastrophic	Concentration camp experience; devastating natural disaster	Multiple family deaths
0	Unspecified	No information, or not applicable	No information, or not applicable

AXIS V: HIGHEST LEVEL OF ADAPTIVE FUNCTIONING PAST YEAR

LEVELS	ADULT EXAMPLES	CHILD OR ADOLESCENT EXAMPLES
1 SUPERIOR Unusually effective functioning in social relations, occupational functioning, and use of leisure time	Single parent living in deteriorating neighborhood takes excellent care of children and home, has warm relations with friends, and finds time for pursuit of hobby.	A 12-year-old girl gets superior grades in school, is extremely popular among her peers, and excels in many sports. She does all of this with apparent ease and comfort.

LEVELS	ADULT EXAMPLES	CHILD OR ADOLESCENT EXAMPLES
2 VERY GOOD Better than average functioning in social relations, occupational functioning, and use of leisure time	A 65-year-old retired widower does some volunteer work, often sees old friends, and pursues hobbies.	An adolescent boy gets excellent grades, works part-time, has several close friends, and plays banjo in a jazz band. He admits to some distress in "keeping up with everything."
3 GOOD No more than slight impairment in either social or occupational functioning	A woman with many friends functions extremely well at a difficult job, but says "the strain is too much."	An 8-year-old boy does well in school, has several friends, but bullies younger children.
4 FAIR Moderate impairment in either social relations or occupational functioning, or moderate impairment in both	A lawyer has trouble carrying through assignments; has several acquaintances, but hardly any close friends.	A 10-year-old girl does poorly in school, but has adequate peer and family relations.

LEVELS	ADULT EXAMPLES	CHILD OR ADOLESCENT EXAMPLES
5 POOR Marked impairment in either social relations or occupational functioning, *or* moderate impairment in both	A man with one or two friends has trouble keeping a job for more than a few weeks.	A 14-year-old boy almost fails in school and has trouble getting along with his peers.
6 VERY POOR Marked impairment in both social relations and occupational functioning	A woman is unable to do any of her housework and has violent outbursts toward family and neighbors.	A 6-year old girl needs special help in all subjects and has virtually no peer relationships.
7 GROSSLY IMPAIRED Gross impairment in virtually all areas of functioning	An elderly man needs supervision to maintain minimal personal hygiene and is usually incoherent.	A 4-year-old boy needs constant restraint to avoid hurting himself and is almost totally lacking in skills.
0 UNSPECIFIED	No information.	No information.